A
Bump
in the
Road

Praise for *A Bump in the Road*

'*A Bump in the Road* is honest, open, raw, emotional and powerful. Elle has shared a story of heartache and hope, and I know her words will be a comfort to others who might feel alone in their struggles. No one should feel isolated by their grief or loss, and with this book Elle has managed to be a hand in the darkness to ensure they aren't. This book isn't only for those who've been through fertility challenges, it's for everyone . . . In this book, once more, her heart is laid bare'

GIOVANNA FLETCHER

'I tore through this beautiful, hopeful book in a couple of days. Elle's fortitude is extraordinary and I'm beyond thrilled that she finally got to write her own happily ever after'

ELLIE TAYLOR

'Another beautiful book, for the many people who are going through this journey. This book gives so much support, hope and strength; a beautiful light at the end of the tunnel. I didn't want to put it down'

JOOLS OLIVER

'A raw and honest account of Elle's journey . . . *A Bump in the Road* reads like a letter from a friend who is pouring their heart out. Full of candour and wit, I have no doubt this heartbreaking but hopeful memoir will offer comfort to a great many women who are facing similar journeys'

SARAH TURNER, THE UNMUMSY MUM

'To see a voice given to some of the feelings many, including me, have experienced after baby loss moved me to tears. This is a book I will pick up again to remind me that pain is as real and valid as hope. A beautifully emotional and healing read, written with the kind of sensitivity that those who have been trying to find hope after baby loss will appreciate'

GENELLE ALDRED

'Heartbreaking yet uplifting . . . I was truly holding my breath'

CAT STRAWBRIDGE, THE FINALLY PREGNANT PODCAST

Praise for *Ask Me His Name*

'It takes a huge amount of courage to re-integrate into the world again after your anticipated version of motherhood has been so brutally and painfully ripped away from you. Yet fuelled by the love of Teddy, Elle has managed to transform her pain into power – becoming a beacon of healing light for all, which is so very much needed in this world'

ANNA LEWIS (SKETCHYMUMA)

'To be able to openly share the unthinkable and write about Teddy with such truth, honesty, beauty and humour takes huge courage. This is such an important book that spoke to me on so many levels – it will give you a deeper understanding about the reality of grief and the true meaning of a mother's love'

IZZY JUDD

'Bold, compelling and heart-wrenchingly honest, this story of how humans can cope in the darkest of hours will blow you away'

MARINA FOGLE

A
Bump
in the
Road

A Story of Fertility,
Hope and Trying Again

Elle Wright

LAGOM

First published in the UK by Lagom
An imprint of Bonnier Books UK
The Plaza, 535 Kings Road, London, SW10 0SZ
Owned by Bonnier Books
Sveavägen 56, Stockholm, Sweden

facebook.com/blinkpublishing
twitter.com/blinkpublishing

Hardback – 978–1–788–703–89–5
Ebook – 978–1–788–703–90–1
Audiobook – 978–1–788–703–91–8

A CIP catalogue of this book is available from the British Library.

Designed by IDSUK (Data Connection) Ltd
Printed and bound by Clays Ltd, Elcograf S.p.A

1 3 5 7 9 10 8 6 4 2

*Elle Wright will donate 1% of all author royalties from the sale of
every book to Tommy's. Bonnier Books UK will also donate 1% of the
published price royalty from the sale of each book to Tommy's.
Tommy's is a registered charity in England and Wales (1060508)
and Scotland (SC039280)*

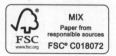

Lagom is an imprint of Bonnier Books UK
www.bonnierbooks.co.uk

For O, because I'd do it all a thousand times over if it led me to you.

And for the doctors, nurses and midwives who were there to hold my hand in delivering the good news and the bad.

They say it takes a village to raise a child. Well, sometimes it takes one to have one too . . .

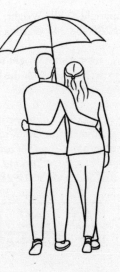

Contents

Foreword

A Note From Emma Cannon,
fertility and women's health expert

FOR MANY, THE ROAD TO PARENTHOOD IS A LONG AND EMOTIONALLY CHALLENGING ONE. So often their pain is poorly understood by those who believe that because they are not ill, they do not suffer. This could not be further from the truth; those who fail to conceive, lose a pregnancy or a child, suffer deeply. However, when we use painful life experiences as a doorway to access our feelings, then healing ourselves is possible. When we share our story with others, we invite them to heal themselves. We turn wounds into wisdom.

Elle's ability to tell her story without the need for victimhood, whilst managing to be the teacher, is extraordinary. The children being born into our new world will need new skills: compassion, curiosity, kindness. When we evolve through our own pain and heal, we change old patterns and we develop the ability to have empathy and compassion for others. These gifts will be passed on to our children. No one wants to suffer. Yet when we allow ourselves to breathe in again, a renewed appreciation for life is born that could not have been reached without our previous experiences.

Longing to conceive comes from the desire to love. It is the greatest human story of all.

Emma Cannon,
October 2020

Introduction

AS I WALKED INTO THE HOSPITAL THAT MORNING, I WAS STRUGGLING TO UNDERSTAND THAT THIS WAS ACTUALLY HAPPENING. *How* could this cruel version of events actually be my reality after already losing my first child, Teddy, at three days old? And yet here I was, back in the hospital delivery suite half a year later to deliver mine and my husband's baby at almost 15 weeks. A baby whose tiny heart had stopped beating a couple of days prior because of some medication I had taken. This was a termination for medical reasons after another heart-breaking diagnosis – something I never imagined I would have to live through, let alone so soon after the death of our son. Yet here we were.

I won't go into the detail of how I delivered that tiny baby, silently, into the world during that first week of January 2017; it's simply too painful to relive. But I will say that it was something that changed my perspective of chasing a 'happy ending' forever. I think this was the moment it dawned on me that this journey to the motherhood I craved so badly was not going to be as straightforward as I had hoped.

The following week, feeling desperate and lonely in my quest to become a mum again, I began writing. This was when my blog was born, and I started to process the emotions I was feeling. It was my form of therapy, a huge cathartic release as those words poured out onto the page. I felt like I was writing more than I would ever publish in my little corner of the internet but it felt too good to stop. A problem shared is a problem halved, as they say. And, as (bad) luck would have it, it turns out there are plenty of us out there – the unlucky ones. The women whose journey into motherhood, or whose yearning for more children, has yet to be fulfilled by the universe. So my writing became a place to tell this story, my motherhood story, in all of its (quite frankly) unbelievably shitty detail.

Then came the opportunity to turn some of my writing about the life of my son Teddy, the pain and grief of losing him, and what life was like for me after, into a book, which I called *Ask Me His Name*.

As teenagers, it seemed we were always being reminded, 'Do not have sex. You *will* get pregnant.' So deep is the belief in our own potent fertility that when we do eventually decide that we are ready to become parents, it's as if we will cast aside that last packet of contraceptive pills and miraculously be 'with child' after no more than a couple of glasses of wine and a romantic weekend away. Even despite the signs our bodies may give us over the years that we might not be the fertile wonder-women that we have been led to believe we are.

I was one who still believed. When we began trying for a baby in 2014, at the age of 29, I truly envisaged that I would blink and be pregnant. Yet I waited a full ten months. A time-frame I now know to be a mere drop in the fertility-fuckery-ocean compared to other people's journeys but one that, nonetheless, broke me with each month of waiting.

It's only now that I realise that perhaps that little stretch was merely a training exercise for the three and a half years we were set to endure after Teddy's death. Years of questions, tests, drugs, procedures, tears, IVF, loss, so many more tears and frustration, all bound together by our shared belief that one day it *would* happen again, somehow.

Now, I am certain that in so many parts of our story, I am not the only one to have gone through it, it makes sense to write it all down. For all of us – and for any women and parents who might go through some of what we did, too.

So here it is in full, our journey to a rainbow. A story of fertility, trying again and, above all, hope.

Chapter 1

Heartbreak and Hopefulness

WHEN WE RETURNED FROM HOSPITAL WITHOUT ANOTHER BABY, I FELT NUMB. That's the best way, the only way, I can describe it. I wondered why it didn't feel as painful as when Teddy had died. Was I in shock? Had I just become accustomed to the pain of heartbreak? Was it that I was comparing losing this baby so much earlier to Teddy dying and feeling like I *couldn't* grieve this loss too? It had only been seven months since Teddy died in May 2016; perhaps I just didn't have space for any more grief. Was I at my grieving capacity, with absolutely no more room for more sadness? All of these questions whirred around in my head leaving me in a heavy fog of confusion and guilt.

Once again, as with the time after we lost Teddy, everyone was kind. The few friends and family we had told before our 12-week scan rushed to comfort us. The hospital and our consultant did what they could to support us with the resources that they had. But I still felt so alone. It just wasn't destined to be 'our time', our 'happy ending' (spoiler alert: I don't think I believe in those anymore).

I tried desperately to pick myself up and dust myself off. I kept thinking, *if I could do it before then* surely *I can do it again?* So, unlike when we were grieving Teddy and trying to give ourselves the time and space to deal with our pain, this time I pushed myself back into 'normal' life. I don't know whether it was a desire for this endless grief to just disappear or a need to feel like myself again. I saw friends around me enjoying their lives and I didn't want to be stuck in this limbo of loss and a feeling of utter hopelessness.

Of course, my attempt to get back to normal too quickly (obviously) caught up with me when I found myself crying in a multi-storey car park after a shopping trip that ended in me crippled with anxiety and needing to get out and get home as quickly as possible. As I sat in the car sobbing, my mum leaned across to hold my hand and told me that we should never have come out, and I knew she was right. Why the fuck I thought shopping was a good idea when I was still bleeding heavily and didn't know what day of the week it was, I shall never know.

As January turned into February I realised that something wasn't quite right with me physically, too. After the initial week of heavy bleeding in January, things had settled down. Then they were back on, and off, and then on again. It was like a tap, one I most certainly wanted to turn off. Each trip to the bathroom was painful reminder that things weren't in fact getting back to normal at all. After a heavy bleed at the end of a yoga class (which I can only describe as a whoosh of excruciating pain and me waddling awkwardly out of the room as quickly as I could muster the power), I was booked for a check-up scan with my consultant. It had been six weeks since we lost the baby and, although the placenta had been delivered in its entirety, she wanted to check on how I was healing.

The scan confirmed my worst fears. There was a bit of the pregnancy that remained lodged in a top corner of my uterus. (First I had heard of a uterus having corners.) My blood tests showed up enough pregnancy hormone to indicate that my body still believed it was pregnant. It explained the persistent bleeding and the heavy head of emotions that I was feeling.

A week later, I was lying on a hospital bed shaking, surrounded by a team of anaesthetists and nurses, waiting to go in for an operation to remove the piece that was causing the problems. I had spent that week using up what must have been all of my remaining positive thoughts in an effort to help it pass naturally. Part of me believed it would; the other part of me was just so crippled with a fear of anaesthetic that I hoped this could all be over before an operation was needed. I remember tears rolling down my cheeks as they put me to sleep. I had a fear of the unknown and a deeper fear that this might cause even further complications and bad luck.

I woke up in recovery a few hours later, heavy-headed and sore beyond belief but relieved it was all over and reassured by my consultant who told me she had been able to get everything out. I felt like I had spent so much time in that hospital in recent months and I just wanted to get home, get into my pyjamas and try to sleep this all off.

In the days that followed, my husband returned to work, my mum came to look after me once more and I realised it was already . . . March?! I had spent the first two months of the year (a year that I had promised myself would be *so* much better than the last) in the middle of a complete nightmare. I wanted to try to make plans again, to be positive and think about trying to pull myself out of this dark hole. The seasons were changing – the blossom was appearing and the bulbs springing up – and I always find it's easier to find optimism at that time of year rather than when we are plunged into the depths of winter.

But all of this new life springing up all around drew my mind back to what I wanted so badly. A new life. I had tried to distract myself, not think about it, give myself a 'few months off' as people suggested.[1] With my body beginning to heal and my next check-up with our consultant just around the corner, I told my husband I wanted to start trying again. Just as after Teddy had died, it wasn't really much of a question or a conversation, more of a mutual agreement that we were in this together and both wanted to do what we could to make this happen. Of course, I knew he was worried about me, about my physical recovery from

---

[1] I can confirm that people who make those 'helpful' suggestions are almost always ones who have never been in the desperate cycle of fertility struggles and loss themselves.

two consecutive losses and the emotional toll that had taken on us both. But he always knew the right thing to say to make me feel as if it was going to be OK, and I hoped I was doing the same for him.

I dusted off the ovulation sticks (by that I obviously mean 'ordered a truckload more from Amazon') and focused on getting myself healthy and fertile. In my mind, as it had happened so quickly (just four short months) after Teddy had been born then it would most certainly happen that way again. I was all set to be expecting again by the summer; all I had to do was *relax* (that old chestnut!), look after myself, pee on sticks at the right time and hope that we had a prevailing wind behind us (as they say). Easy. I felt like I knew what I was doing with this trying-to-conceive lark now. I was a seasoned pro.

Wrong.

Three months passed and I barely had a period. Well, not one that I would say 'counted' – it was a fleeting day at best. Obviously, after the first month when it was late and then barely there, I convinced myself that I was pregnant again. Only to be confused by every negative test. The next month was like a cruel repeat of the first and so on . . . This had to be some kind of joke, right? In January and February my body didn't seem to be able to stop bleeding – and now this? I began to worry. I'd had times in my life before – in my early twenties, when my weight had dropped, I had been working too hard, stressing too much and my periods had disappeared – so I knew it could happen. But now? When I needed my body to be on my team and working how I needed it to. *Really?*

I contacted my consultant and asked for another follow-up; as everything had looked back to normal at my early April scan, she had been expecting me to be three cycles into normality by now. She arranged for me to have a hysteroscopy as soon as possible. I'm happy to admit that when I first read the letter I definitely read it as 'hysterectomy' and thought she was being a little hasty, but quickly realised it was just an investigative procedure where they pop a camera up there and have a bit of a rummage around (technical terms, obviously) to see if they can find anything that isn't being picked up on a scan. It does, however, need to be done at a certain time in your cycle, which seemed an impossible task as mine had all but disappeared. They allowed me to go on guess-work and two weeks later I was there with legs up in stirrups while a very kind nurse held my hand and assured me it would be over in no time. BLOODY HELL. I thought after childbirth it might be a walk in the park, perhaps no more painful than a cervical screening? Incorrect. The consultant who performed it was also kind and very apologetic for the pain she was causing, and I found myself thanking everyone in the room in a terribly awkward and British way upon exiting.

When I returned to see my consultant at the end of June, she assured me that the results of the hysteroscopy had come back normal. There was nothing else hanging around in there that could be upsetting the feng shui. So, I was met with the infamous internal scanner once more. One of my friends who had also experienced complications and loss once casually referred to the scanner as 'the dildo wand', an analogy that has remained firmly in my mind forevermore and caused borderline sniggering whenever I was presented with another encounter with this tool.

Upon inspection, everything looked normal – 'normal but quiet', I heard the consultant say. She explained that my ovaries were presenting polycystically, which meant I had no main follicle from which to release a mature egg each month, and instead had lots of little ones just hanging around in there not doing much. Staring blankly at the screen, taking in all of those useless little dots that were doing absolutely bugger all for our chances of conceiving again, I felt a swell of sadness rising up within me. Before I knew it or could stop it, my eyes were burning and hot, and heavy tears were streaming down my face.

'I'm sorry. I'm sorry,' I kept repeating, as I sat there firmly believing I was the only woman to have ever lost her composure in the midst of being told her chances of conception right now were slim-to-none. Of course, the consultant had seen it all before. She was kind, patient, understanding and promised me that we would get to the bottom of what was happening in there and why. I believed her and I thanked her. I was beginning to feel more confused than ever and grew weary of not knowing what was going on in there, but I trusted she would help me as best she could. Which made me feel a little less desperate, given the circumstances.

I would visit again the following month at a time she expected to be my mid-cycle point. In the meantime, I was set to have bloods taken before (guessed time of) ovulation, and again afterwards to see if it had occurred. I felt happy with this plan but it didn't seem to solve the case of the missing periods – by this point I had never yearned for a period more in my life. I asked her why I wasn't bleeding properly and she explained that it might be a hormonal imbalance caused by lack of ovulation, or perhaps due to all of the stress and confusion my body had been through over the past year. I had to admit, it wasn't surprising that my ovaries and womb had gone on strike. I think I'd have shut up shop by now if I were them. I was also pretty sure they picked that attitude up from me, given how the last year had panned out. I was referred to another doctor at the hospital to have an HSG (hysterosalpingogram) procedure to see if there was any obstruction in my fallopian tubes. Surely those guys hadn't given up on me too?

Despite the delivery of this less-than-ideal news, as I walked out of the hospital alone that day into the June sunshine, we had a plan. I felt a real glimmer of optimism for the first time in a long time.

Chapter 2

Things Can Only Get Better

AS THE SUMMER ROLLED ON, MORE TESTS, APPOINT-MENTS AND CHECK-UPS AT THE HOSPITAL BECAME A REGULAR FEATURE OF LIFE. I was having monthly blood tests to monitor ovulation. These were performed at different times in my cycle to try to detect both a rise in LH – or luteinising hormone – which indicates ovulation is imminent, and a potential rise of progesterone post-ovulation. Each time my GP called to tell me that neither were really detectable. Perhaps my ovaries, as suspected, had indeed shut up shop?

A particular highlight of this investigatory period was the HSG procedure. I had heard a few people refer to it as a 'flushing of the tubes', which made me shudder at the very thought of it. It's designed to detect blockages or adhesions in the fallopian tubes that could be causing fertility complications. Essentially, anything in there that could potentially be stopping a healthy egg from travelling on its merry way to the uterus so that the wonder of conception could happen. I think this was the only procedure that I felt genuinely nervous about. Not only because of the military precision at which point in the cycle it had to be performed, but because it might show up something else; another challenge that we weren't expecting.

Nico came with me to the hospital that day. It was a sweltering summer's day and I remember sitting in the waiting room, clammy-handed and visibly shaking with apprehension. When I was called in to the room, I won't pretend my face wasn't agog with shock when it became apparent that the consultant performing the procedure was a man, who seemed not too dissimilar in age to me. He read my expression and hurriedly explained he was covering a patient list for a colleague that day. Feeling guilty about the face I had obviously pulled, I then instantly felt more anxiety for him than I did for myself. I'm by no means shy nor easily embarrassed, so I tried to make light of the situation with a few jokes along the lines of: '*Well, pretty much everyone else at the hospital has had a look down there now, you may as well join the club!*' I'm really not sure if I made things less awkward or more.

There were several nurses on hand, all with kind faces and genuine empathy for the situation that I was facing, and I climbed up onto the bed and assumed the frog position ready for inspection. I remember one of them offering me her hand, saying, 'You can squeeze as hard as you like. This might be a little painful.' The consultant was brilliant and he continued to chat to me and tried to put me at ease throughout. It was obvious he had read my notes beforehand too, as he explained how very sorry he was to hear about Teddy and told me about his friends who had lost a child in similar circumstances.

The procedure itself lasted about 15–20 minutes. It involved injecting a fluid dye up into the uterine cavity that sort of blasts (probably the wrong word to use there) up through the fallopian tubes. He turned the screens on so I could watch too as they monitored the fluid by ultrasound travelling along. It was painful – a strange stinging and cramping pain that I wasn't expecting – but it was brief and I knew it would get us some more answers as to what was going on in there.

As I climbed off the bed and was preparing to scuttle back behind the curtain and regain what little of my dignity I had left by replacing my hospital gown with clothing once more, the consultant asked if I could just sit up and have a quick chat for a moment. I feared it might be bad news and froze. His face softened and looked understanding; I think he could read the desperation in my eyes and wanted to put me out of my misery. He said, 'Now I don't want you to be going home and wasting any more energy worrying about this, so I will just tell you now that everything looks normal to me.' A moment of sheer joy. 'As far as I can see, there are no issues with your tubes. No blockages, no evidence of anything that shouldn't be there.'

My legs were shaking as I stepped down from the bed. I'm not sure if it was the position I had assumed, the shock of a good result or the knowledge that yet another roomful of people had been staring between my legs for best part of half an hour, but my legs felt as though they were about to give way. I walked slowly and unsteadily to get changed, thanking everyone as I did so. As I emerged again into the room, the same consultant said goodbye with a cheery smile and wished me well. I could tell he meant it too.

I staggered back into the waiting room to the smiling face of my husband. 'All OK?' he asked, concern showing on his face as he saw me wincing with each step.

'Surprisingly, yes.'

'Was it painful?'

'Fucking awful. Can we go home now please?'

The rest of the afternoon passed with a shower, some snack foods (because they solve everything) and a nap. I felt relieved; for now, at least, we weren't dealing with anything else. I knew so many women who were. Through my writing and social media, I had begun, tentatively, to share parts of our trying-to-conceive-again-after-loss (catchy title) journey and had already connected with so many wonderful women who were already openly sharing their trials and tribulations of trying for a baby. I must admit that it had opened my eyes to so many gynaecological issues that I hadn't even considered when we had innocently stumbled into the world of trying for a baby almost two years previously. I was becoming educated in all of the potential challenges that couples can face and, more importantly, overcome when trying for a family. I felt like I had a safety net of support. Blogs to read, podcasts to listen to. It was like discovering the 'loss world' post-Teddy all over again. After he died, suddenly this huge chasm opened and I was dropped into an existence I hadn't ever been aware of; all of these mothers, just like me, the unlucky ones. A world I never knew existed but that would soon become such a huge support, lifeline even, for me.

A few weeks later, my next visit to the consultant was, again, a positive one. After the discomfort and shock of the HSG, I had been riding on the high of knowing that my fallopian tubes had a clean bill of health (always looking for the positives) and felt almost certain that it wouldn't be long before those ovaries would wake up and we would be back on track to baby-making.

As she went over the results of my tests, the consultant agreed that everything looked clear. She then went over my blood test results that still seemed to show no rise in hormones at either stage in my cycles. With my periods still barely there, she performed another internal scan. There they were, the quiet ovaries. She explained that the little follicles were still there, that there were (likely) no dominant follicles forming each month to release a healthy egg. In other words, even if the eggs were there, busting to come out, they had no transport to their required destination. In that moment I felt deflated and defeated once more. The lining of my uterus, which at this late point in my cycle should have been a good thickness (plump and ripe, ready to house any potential fertilised embryo wishing to bed-in for the long haul), was thin. It didn't seem surprising to her that I wasn't having a monthly cycle given these circumstances.

So, what to do now? We went over everything again: my diet, did I smoke, my weight, anything else that could have been causing it. There was, of course, one common denominator here – stress. In my desperation to become pregnant again after losing Teddy and then the subsequent heartbreak of another lost little one, I had become extremely focused on my one goal: getting pregnant again. I had put all of my metaphorical eggs in one basket, obsessing over this as the one thing I needed to achieve, and of course, my body had been pushed to its limits already. It had decided that it wasn't ready.

I recall her asking me if I wanted to try to do anything now to try to help things along a little. She had barely finished her sentence before I found myself replying all too hastily, 'Yes, please. Anything. I'll try anything.' Ahhh, the words of a desperate woman, and I knew she could read it on my face. As I twisted and turned a tissue over and over between my tense fingers, holding back the stinging tears that were rising once more, I listened intently as she explained what the next steps might be. The options were all backed up with anatomical pictures on sheets that detailed how we might get things working again. It was like a science lesson for the infertile.

The consultant was reluctant to put me on any kind of ovulation-induction drug until we had tried a softer approach. I appreciated her methodical approach, I didn't want to jump head-first into fertility drugs either. After all, my body had done this before, twice! Surely we could remind it what to do again? I felt optimistic and I had to take that chance. The first suggested treatment was a form of hormone therapy, a little like HRT given to women experiencing the menopause. It seemed simple enough: oestrogen patches for the first two weeks of my cycle, stuck to somewhere fleshy and discreet like a bum or a leg and changed every few days. Then again in the second two weeks but now accompanied by daily progesterone tablets to mimic the second phase of a natural cycle. The oestrogen was designed to help build the uterus lining and encourage an LH surge and, in turn, ovulation; the progesterone would support the second part of the cycle and encourage either a pregnancy to be achieved or the cycle to end and a period to begin again naturally each month.

It was a gentle approach, it seemed logical and I welcomed it. All of the logic seemed to have been dispelled from my brain in recent months, replaced by panic and desperation to be pregnant. The focus of this course of medication would be to restore my cycles, not just with the sole intention of becoming pregnant again. The consultant issued me with a prescription and an instruction of when to begin, booked me in for a review appointment after another couple of months, and off I went – clutching my prescription and a new-found glimmer of hope. Before I walked out of the room she said, 'And don't forget to do your homework. So many couples waiting for medical intervention don't do that you know.' She smiled and I sniggered and replied, 'Yes, of course.' It felt strange for my doctor to be instructing me to go home and have sex with my husband. I knew what she meant: keep on trying and don't think it won't happen. Even when it appears that the odds are stacked against you.

Once I had started my medication, I decided to double-down on my own efforts to give my body its best chance of recuperation. There were definitely things I could be doing and I didn't want to be reliant on medication to be a magic wand in all of this. I knew if I went into this with a healthy approach then I could say I did everything I possibly could to make it work. I had already been having acupuncture to help with fertility, something I had begun in the months after Teddy had died. It had been a lifeline in helping me to recover after the loss of our last baby too. Not just physically, but emotionally. It helped me to sleep and allowed my fractious mind to calm. The only way I could describe its effects would be to say it was like taking all of those thoughts and feelings – anxiety, worry, grief and everything in between – and arranging them all neatly in some kind of order in a filing cabinet in my mind. Allowing me still to sit with all of those feelings but not bury them. To just be able to feel them and address them with a more organised approach, without feeling that constant rise of panic in my chest. Each time I had treatment, I no longer walked around with those constant feelings of overwhelming grief and confusion caused by the events of the last 18 months. I felt freer somehow.

I began reading up on other forms of Chinese medicine, nutrition and diet – ways in which I could nourish my body. The teachings of Chinese medicine attribute a lot of our fertility concerns to the way we eat and treat ourselves, and to our body and blood type. I found it fascinating. It was then that I stumbled across someone who was about to become a huge support and inspiration, but I didn't know I would be lucky enough to one day also call her a friend.

When I first saw Emma Cannon's *Fertile* book spring up on my Amazon suggested reads, I was nothing short of intrigued. It was a word I looked for, clung to and so desperately wanted to feel within me. It had just been published, her most recent in a long line of books, all born out of a lifetime of dedication to Chinese medicine and treating women to help them achieve their dream of motherhood. It was the easiest 'Buy Now' that I ever clicked on.

I devoured most of the book a few days later whilst sitting on a beach in Cornwall, each page filling me with a delight about finally becoming an expert in *my own* fertility. Emma is focused and passionate about empowering women to believe in their own body's ability and believe in themselves. Her book aims to teach us to focus on our own paths and trust that it will get us to exactly where we need to be. To not become consumed by what others are achieving, especially when it comes to fertility and having babies.

It can come to be seen as a race, a competition even, and it's all too easy to become distracted by how many babies others seem to be so easily popping out into this world when all you long for is just one to take home.

I began following Emma on Instagram and read her posts with the eagerness of a child who was learning something brand new. I also began to change my diet, but I wouldn't say that happened overnight. I tried not to stick to anything with great rigidity (as we all know, this adds a different kind of pressure). I knew I needed to eat more protein where I could and cut down on things that might thin my uterine lining or stop my ovaries from functioning properly. I cut out caffeine and cut down on alcohol. I hadn't really been drinking after Teddy died anyway as I was too scared of feeling out of control. I suppose I feared it might let my emotions run wild, and not in a good way; it's a depressant, after all. At this point limiting myself to one, maybe two drinks a week was no change at all. I learned that I was cold-blooded and needed to nourish myself with hot soups and stews, take warm baths and time to enjoy the sunshine (not always easy in the UK, I know). It was a revelation, a focus away from just 'getting pregnant again' and instead on regaining control of my own body, my natural cycle and truly understanding how my body was working.

After engaging with what Emma posted on her social media, I was surprised to see a message from her pop up in my inbox one day. She explained that someone I knew had been to her clinic and told her about me, Teddy and the struggles we had been experiencing since. She said she just wanted to reach out, to send some love and positivity my way. I replied explaining that I had been reading her latest book and what a positive impact it had already had on me (more mentally at this point than anything). She explained that she also had a clinic treating patients in London and although she had practitioners who saw a lot of her patients, that if I were ever to book, she would love to see me and treat me herself. Needless to say, later that week I booked myself an appointment for a consultation.

I couldn't wait to hear her diagnosis of what I needed. I yearned for that kind of positive emotional support and not just medical intervention. The hormone treatment was working; I was one cycle in and experiencing more of a period than I had ever had in recent months. Small steps, but steps in the right direction. I waited for my appointment with Emma in anticipation of what else I might learn.

She didn't disappoint. After meeting with her, I knew her approach would be something that would not only help me but keep me going through this. At the end of the appointment, she said something to me that I will never forget, something no one else had dared ask me to this point, something no one had questioned. She looked at me and calmly said, 'Elle, why do you want another baby?'

I was dumbstruck. I couldn't believe the words that had just left her mouth. My son had died and I suppose I thought it might have been pretty obvious, to anyone, why I wanted another baby. Or was it? I could tell she read the bewilderment on my face with ease.

'What do you mean?' I replied. She knew what thoughts were going through my head, that I longed to be a mother again to a baby who came home this time. But she wanted me to say it and see it for myself.

'Each time you are struggling, losing focus, feeling lost, I want you to close your eyes, put a hand on your heart and one on your belly and ask yourself why you want another baby.'

As she spoke, I began to do just that and the words came tumbling out. I wanted to regain that sense of motherhood, fill that void of purposeless that had been created when Teddy left us. I wasn't looking to replace him, I was just longing to hold another little human into whom we could pour all of this love, love that felt like it had no place to go.

I said those words aloud for Emma to hear and she simply nodded and smiled. 'Then remember that.'

We hugged and I thanked her. I felt renewed, walking on air. Clutching a copy of another of her books, I left her office and skipped down the road like a scene from a fucking musical. I hadn't felt this empowered about anything in I didn't know how long. I had become lost in this process already, I was quickly losing myself again, but this had pulled me back. I could see now. Things could only get better. Couldn't they?

Chapter 3

Metformin & Me

THE NEXT MONTH OR SO PASSED WITH ME ENJOYING MY NEW-FOUND LOVE OF INVESTING IN MY OWN FERTILITY. I know it sounds desperately clichéd and, dare I say, a little cheesy but I was feeling less lost in all of this and more 'me' than I had in a while. I was finally able to plan things again, to see friends and learn to enjoy things a little more. My appointment with my consultant couldn't come soon enough as I was keen to see if my efforts were beginning to pay off physiologically. I wanted to know if she could see anything different when she looked at scans; if my blood test results would be any different. Basically, I just wanted to know if anything I was doing was making the smallest impact on my body. I had continued on the hormone treatment and, to be fair, I hadn't experienced any of the side effects she had warned about. I didn't know if this was a good sign or not: maybe not feeling anything meant it wasn't working? I tried not to dwell on it too much.

It was early October by the time this next appointment to 'check progress' rolled around. Weirdly, I felt excited to know exactly what that progress looked like. I was hooked and starting to understand that the fertility world is a strange and powerful vortex that sucks you in. Monitoring everything, checking for signs and symptoms, what-ifs. It was a cruel mistress and I was very much under its spell, swinging from hope to hopelessness in a heartbeat. Waiting for my body to respond in the way I wanted it to, given all of the weird and wonderful things I was doing to help it along the way.

My consultant was always wonderfully matter-of-fact in our meetings, giving it to me straight and never sugar-coating the situation. I know that might not be how some people like news to be delivered, but it suited me down to the ground. I was there for the facts. As she began scanning, her face looked mildly hopeful (although I must say, I have always marvelled at what great poker faces all medical professionals have).

'Well, your lining looks a little thicker. Which is good.' Tick, first positive bit of news that I felt like I had heard in a while.

'But your ovaries, still quiet. I am still not sure if you are ovulating each month and your bloods would indicate that too.' Fuck. Back down to Earth with a bump. Mother Nature, she giveth and then she taketh away.

'What does this mean?' I asked, shimmying back into my jeans and feeling like I was once again staring at her with my wide-eyed, pleading look of '*Please tell me we have another card to play?*'

'The hormone treatment seems to be working but I'd like to try it alongside another drug. Hopefully it will get your ovaries kick-started again. It's often used as a drug for diabetes, it's called metformin.'

A drug for diabetes? Nothing made sense anymore but I was prepared to give it a whirl. At this point, actually, I felt like I was prepared to give anything a whirl. Had she said, 'Well I think it's a great idea to set yourself on fire and run down the street naked,' I'd probably have taken a moment to consider my options . . .

She explained that metformin could help the way my body regulated its blood sugar and that this was often linked to improving the function of the ovaries, particularly in women whose ovaries behaved polycystically or who had suffered long-term with PCOS. For some, it worked brilliantly; in others it might not do anything at all, but it was worth exploring. It was something that had to be started on a relatively low dose so I began with one tablet a day (with food) and after some time I worked up to three tablets a day. One possible drawback, and the reason I was to increase my dosage gradually, was the side effects. Nausea, diarrhoea, upset stomach, headaches, weight loss . . . Oh boy, I couldn't *wait* to give this a try! Like I said, I didn't care, anything was worth a shot.

It had been ten (long) months since our last loss. We had spent ten months trying for Teddy, then four months had passed after losing him before we fell pregnant again, meaning we had officially hit the three-year mark of trying for a baby and there still being no baby at home. Since losing Teddy, I had lost count of the number of friends who had already become pregnant again. People who had been planning families at the same time as us now already had one baby in the bank and another one on the way. Why wasn't that us? I tried my best not to get too caught up in the frustration of it all, in the months and the years and the calendar rolling over each time with no success.

Metformin was obviously going to be the answer to all of our wishes, wasn't it? The first few weeks felt easy enough; there were no real side effects that I could feel. It seemed to be OK taking it with the hormones I was already on. I kept taking my usual vitamins alongside everything too and was one step off rattling when I walked. I upped my dosage of metformin after three weeks to two tablets a day. No problem. Well, maybe the odd headache and a bit of a bad tummy but that could be down to normal cyclical changes anyway. Was I losing weight? It's difficult to tell when you see yourself in the mirror each and every day, isn't it? A few of my clothes felt looser but, to be fair, I had been a fair few pounds heavier since I had Teddy, so perhaps this was just my body finally returning to its pre-pregnancy size.

November came, I upped my dosage again: three tablets now. I wasn't due for another progress check until January so I wanted to at least make sure I had given my best effort to making this drug work.

'Bloody hell, you've lost weight!'

These words echoed in my ears as a friend greeted me during a pre-Christmas catch up.

'Yeah, must be all that yoga, eh?' I was talking utter bollocks in a desperate attempt to keep the conversation as far away from fertility chat as possible. I didn't have the energy. All my friends were kind, so kind, and trying their very best to sensitively ask me how things were going in that department. But so often, like after Teddy had died, I found myself feeling utterly exhausted explaining the ins and outs of fertility to them and the workings of the combination of drugs I had been put on.

Another thing I found with metformin was that even my weekly (sometimes bi-weekly) glass of wine made me feel fucking awful. Like I'd been on a weekend bender reminiscent of the previous decade. Not worth the headache, literally. So, yes, I was looking gaunt and the relaxing pleasure of a weekend glass of vino had also been removed from the equation. But I was *bound* to get pregnant. Right?

I didn't know if metformin was working or not. I was pretty sure the other hormone drugs were still doing their thing – since beginning them in the summer I had now experienced three (yes *three*) almost-periods. I say 'almost' as these were still two-to-three days of not much action at all but they were there, so things were on the up. I was eating as many blood-nourishing foods as I could in an attempt to improve things. Spinach and kale, cherries and dates, downing beetroot juice like it was going out of fashion. Can I just say, I fucking hate beetroot juice. There, glad that's out in the open. I said to my mum at the time, 'When this is all over, I pledge never to drink another glass of beetroot juice as long as I live. I don't care if it cures cancer. It turns my mouth pink and tastes like I am literally licking soil.' The end. That said, it's supposed to be great for improving blood flow to your uterus and helps in creating a healthy lining, both things I needed, so I persevered with the disgusting beetroot juice.

However, my acupuncturist, who I had been seeing since our last loss and my operation to remove retained tissue from that pregnancy, had mostly been telling me that things had felt 'lifeless' in there. Brilliant. All my efforts and still no life to be found. It was at this point, at the end of 2017, that a friend recommended I also tried Chinese herbs alongside acupuncture. She had used them with great success and was expecting again after her own loss and a complicated journey of IVF. She explained how they had been prescribed just for her and designed to support her treatment. Another thing to throw into the mix? Sure, why not.

The following month, I skipped off to my first consultation with her practitioner. That Christmas had been our second without Teddy, still not expecting, and willing to try anything. It's weird but when I look at photos of that Christmas, of me standing in the kitchen at my parents' house and grinning next to my mum, I can see that my mouth is smiling but my eyes look hollow. My face is gaunt and I look tired, visibly exhausted from desperately trying to put on a brave face for 19 months. I look almost painfully thin from the effects of metformin and my Christmas Day dress hangs from my frame. I am merrily clutching a glass of champagne (that I recall not even finishing). What others see in a photo and what we see ourselves can tell two very different stories. Trying something new, like Chinese herbs, felt like a good way to bolster my mood in January. A positive start to the year. Something else I could say I had tried before my next check-in at the hospital.

The lady who greeted me wasn't who I expected at all. Perhaps 15 years older than me (at the very most), she had beautiful long, strawberry-blonde hair and a smiling face. She explained that she had, in fact, trained with Emma Cannon. My faith in her grew ten-fold in that moment. My consultation lasted about an hour and there were tears. I had to tell her everything, from losing Teddy to where we were now. My mum came with me for moral support as I couldn't face telling another stranger the sorry tale of it all on my own. I needed someone who could interject in case I couldn't speak, and no one knew the full story like her. It was also really handy having my mum there as the practitioner was able to ask her questions about her own fertility experiences and births. Having had three of us, my mum is fairly well versed in the world of making babies and happily answered all of the questions posed. It is said, in Chinese practice, that we inherit much of our fertility tendencies and traits from our mothers. Once the consultation was over (which included looking at my tongue and listening to my pulse), she asked if I would like to have some quick needling done while she prepared my herb prescription. She continued chatting to my mum while I lay there and waited for the needles in my tummy, arms and head to work their magic. It felt incredibly calm and safe in her practice room and I trusted that whatever she was prescribing would be right for me.

It turns out that Chinese medicine in the UK is much like conventional medicine, in that you can't just go casually buying it over the counter. You have to have a prescription and then that prescription has to be checked and sent by a regulated distributor of Chinese medicines. I wasn't able to go skipping out of the room that day with my new-fangled herbal prescription, I had to wait for them to arrive by post. She warned me that they might be strange at first, awful to taste and not very palatable. They were designed to boost each stage of my cycle and give my body what it was lacking.

There were four parts to the prescription: sachets to be taken during the days of my period, different ones for the following days leading up to ovulation, then further sachets to be taken for three days over the predicted ovulation days (I say 'predicted' because I was playing it pretty fast and loose at this point as to whether my body had regained its ability to do this) and lastly sachets for the 'two-week wait' (a time-frame that those trying to conceive a baby will be only too familiar with). For anyone lucky enough not to be familiar with, or indeed dread this wonderful time, I'm referring to the two weeks after you ovulate in your cycle, where you wish, hope, pray (and any other form of positive thinking!) that you might just get a second line appear on that test when you finally take it at the end of those weeks.

These last ones were supposed to boost the environment in which fertilisation and implantation might take place. They weren't even herbs like I had envisaged they might be; they were brown granules. Not dissimilar to instant coffee in appearance but tasting, well, absolutely bloody awful. Utterly vile, truth be told. It was everything I could do to keep them down, once dissolved in their recommended amount of warm water and hastily downed with nose held tightly in a vain attempt to keep the taste at bay.

By this point, I am pretty certain friends and family thought I had gone mad. My husband's face tuned to sheer disgust when I got him to so much as sniff the contents of each delightful potion. 'That looks like pond water,' was his horrified verdict. I'm pretty sure it didn't taste far off either. I wanted to keep at it though. I had arranged a second visit to the Chinese medicine practitioner in March and I wanted to have made it through my first prescription.

Later that month, my hospital check-in appointment rumbled around once more. These were becoming a regular feature of despair and delight in my calendar.

There were points at which I felt like I spoke to or saw either my consultant or her secretary more often than many of my friends. It wasn't even a feeling, it was a fact. I barely had to utter the word hello and the secretary knew exactly who was speaking. I became increasingly paranoid that each time I called or chased correspondence, she pitied me or my perseverance was becoming an annoyance. I felt like a desperate woman, chasing each appointment, each blood result, each tiny glimmer of hope.

This time, there just *had* to be good news. I had been on metformin for four months and I was literally a shadow of my former self. The extra hormones had been coursing around my body for nearly seven months now. I was (almost) five periods in. You could have heard a pin drop when she was scanning. I am pretty sure I actually held my breath.

'I don't think the metformin is doing anything for you on its own.'

Tears. I could feel them pricking at my eyes again. *Please don't cry*, I pleaded to myself, *not while she's still got that bloody wand up there*. As I climbed off the bed once more and prepared to sit at her desk for the 'So, what next?' chat, I could feel myself beginning to panic. What exactly *were* the next steps?

She explained precisely what she saw. My ovaries appeared with fewer small follicles on. This was good news, but although there were fewer, there were still multiple small ones, meaning no dominant follicle; bad news. In order to ovulate, you need a dominant follicle to release an egg at any given time of the month; and my body still didn't seem to be achieving this. My bloods had been varied – one cycle I might have ovulated, the others it didn't look likely. My lining was increasing but still not as thick or as healthy as it might have been before all of this began. So, where the hell did that leave us?

'Before we look into the possibility of assisted fertility treatment like IUI or IVF, I think it would be a good idea to try a drug called clomiphene – known to most as Clomid.'

Forget anything else she said in that sentence because every detail went over my head. Apart from three letters: IVF. What the actual fuck? Why was she mentioning IVF? My head began to pound, my palms were sweating, my heart felt like it might explode out of my chest. Why does she think we need to have IVF? I was panicking that things were worse than she had let on, but they couldn't be, she had always been so straight to the point. At this point, the consultant sensed my panic that we were heading into a realm of discussion that I hadn't been prepared for.

'I'm not saying you'll need IVF; many couples don't get that far. There are other things we can try before we get there. It's good to know there are options and that IVF would be the last thing we would try. For now, I think clomiphene is the next logical step.'

The facts about Clomid (as the drug is called) were pretty simple. You take it from days two to six of your cycle and it urges your ovary to produce a dominant follicle from which to release an egg. Simple. As with everything, there were potential side effects. Headaches and nausea, some women become irritable, have mood swings, can even feel depressed or manic. Lastly, Clomid can reduce the thickening of the lining, meaning periods could become lighter, so it wasn't designed to be used for more than six cycles. I could try it from February to August (allowing seven months instead of six, as my scanty cycles were longer and unpredictable).

The plan was to cut my metformin dosage right down to just one tablet a day and keep on the oestrogen patches. I would then add in the Clomid when my next period came (due any day after this appointment). It was a lot to take in but I was confident that we hadn't rushed to this point. Besides, time was ticking on. It was over a year since we had lost our last baby. We were three and a half months away from Teddy's second birthday. Why *was* time going so quickly? Or was it that I had been sucked so far into this fertility vortex that now the months, the years even, were whizzing past in a haze as we clawed at ways to make this work?

I left with another prescription in hand. A list of drugs as long as my arm. I walked out of the hospital clutching paper bags full of neatly packed pills and patches, enough to last me the next few months. My next check-in was booked for April. We would likely know if anything was working by then.

When my husband came home that evening, I updated him on the days goings-on and the details of my latest appointment. I took him though the packs of pills and what I was due to take and when.

'Elle, this is all getting a bit much, isn't it?'

His main concern was if I really was OK to be carrying on down this road, pumping my body full of drugs in the hope that it might make a dream come true for us both. The truth is, I didn't know, but I knew after the investigations and tests that I was already beginning to carry the weight of knowing that this was (most likely) *my* problem. It was my body that wasn't playing ball and was preventing this from happening for us again, and therefore my burden to shoulder. I felt as though it was my duty, that I owed it to us both to do my very best here. Take the drugs, look after myself, eat well, don't drink, keep downing the Chinese herbs, the list went on and on.

'I won't tell you that she mentioned IVF then . . .'

His face was as ashen as I suspected mine had been at the clanging of those three letters in the consultant's office. Funny really, we all know what they mean (or at least we think we do) but none of us really appreciates the magnitude of those letters or what that process might involve until they are posed to us in a sentence that involves our own future.

'It's OK. It's not imminent,' I said before he could reply. 'It's just on the radar, as an option. We have options, this is good.'

Options. I was right, we did have options. Lots of them. We were only a very short distance down a very long path. Not near the end, or even nearing the end. There were so many things we could do, that could happen, before we came anywhere near running out of options. I think I already knew at this point that I was prepared to try all of them.

Chapter 4

Just Do IVF

I WATCHED AS HER TEASPOON SWIRLED IN THE MUG
AND THE WORDS FELL OUT OF HER MOUTH BEFORE
SHE COULD COMPREHEND THEIR MEANING: 'It's all
very well taking these next steps, but you're putting
your body through so much medication. Why can't
you just do IVF?'

Well-meaning pep-talks from friends were becoming
a regular occurrence. Wise words, usually given while
they bounced a baby on their knee or chased a restless
toddler around the room.

Or, 'Have you thought about adoption?'

No. No to both. For now, at least. You see, with
all the best will in the world, it's never going to be as

simple as just *doing* IVF. The very suggestion made it sound as though I might saunter into my consultant's office, slide my ticket across the desk and say eagerly, 'One for IVF, please.'

I felt as if I had spent the last (almost) two years of my life trying to educate friends in the reality of child-loss and now had been tasked with explaining again and again the intricacies of fertility investigations and treatment plans. All the while, people were effort-lessly procreating around me and asking us why we didn't just pursue IVF straight away or adopt a baby? Did they just want a quick fix to the problem or were they genuinely trying to help me? I tried my hardest to believe the latter and bit my tongue through so many of those conversations.

It was going to be a long time before most of us un-derstood the magnitude of committing to IVF treat-ment or the time-frame and tick-lists that needed to be completed before you are even considered eligible for it. You see, even if we had just wanted to sign up there and then, and simply requested to do IVF, there were roads that would have to have been travelled first. First of all there needs to have been a minimum of two years of trying, unsuccessfully, to fall pregnant naturally. Then an investigation into possible causes of fertility complications, which includes scans, blood tests, hysteroscopy, HSG, sperm testing. Other methods to assist conception are then tried: hormones, metformin and now Clomid (generally seen as the last chance saloon before the letters IUI and IVF become regular features in conversations). We only realised all of these things ourselves once we were in the 'system'.

Even someone with the money to seek treatment privately would still need to meet these criteria in the eyes of most practising fertility doctors, unless (as I understand) age and time were a particularly pressing matter, which, for us, as I was not yet 33 at this point, neither were. All of these bridges needed to be crossed before we would be coming close to IVF. Then it would be the next logical step, the only logical step.

When I mentioned this to friends, it would often be greeted with, 'And how do you feel about that?'

'Fucking terrified to be honest. I didn't think it would come to that.'

I had to be honest, there was no point in sugar-coating it to make things more palatable for others. It's not a course of action I was in a hurry to pursue, no matter how desperate I felt. The truth was, I wanted this whole problem to disappear, to be sitting there happily bouncing a baby on my knee like they were. For now,

I felt trapped on this road, trying to keep my focus on what lay ahead instead of becoming distracted by what I saw around me and the 'helpful suggestions' that came in droves, often from people who had seemingly never faced any fertility complications in their lives. Strange how someone who fell pregnant so easily might think telling me to put my legs in the air after sex or to 'just use ovulation sticks, you'll get pregnant' would be helpful or brand-new information. Not if you're not fucking ovulating you won't . . . Sometimes a blunt response in a jovial manner was all I could muster to shut down the 'helpfulness'. My friends were understanding, they knew when I'd had enough fertility chat for one day. I knew it all came from a good place, a place of people wanting to say something to help, but when you're the one still sitting there empty-armed as they cheerfully knock back a glass of rosé over the sleeping infant in their arms, you can't help but feel like screaming. (Or crying. Perhaps both?)

So, Clomid it was. We were in round one and it seemed to be going well. I mean, I *had* experienced some of the symptoms I'd be warned of: headaches, hot flushes and my skin was breaking out like never before. But it

wasn't *terrible* . . . I also had an unquenchable thirst –
no amount of water I drank seemed to solve it.

Before starting Clomid, I had been settling into
29–33(ish)-day cycles and my (almost) periods once
more. I was convinced that one round of this stuff and
I'd be expecting again. I continued the acupuncture,
followed Emma's eating plans, practised yoga daily
and kept on downing those awful Chinese herbs. I
was feeling so optimistic we even booked a holiday.
We hadn't been away anywhere since our honeymoon
four years previously and we were fast approaching
two years since Teddy died. Booking something fun,
something to look forward to away from all of this,
felt like the right thing to do. We booked a week in
Dubai the following month, April 2018, and I couldn't
wait. It felt like a dream come true that we could finally afford a holiday again after pouring all of our
money into house renovations for the past three and
a half years. Part of me was even convinced I would
be pregnant by then and this whole sorry tale would
be over.

It was mid-March and my first cycle of Clomid
would be coming to an end over the next two weeks.
I awaited my period, kept calm, focused on writing
Ask Me His Name, and tried not to think about what

the end of the cycle would bring. My period didn't come – not after 28 days and not after 33. Should I test? I didn't dare. I had been using ovulation sticks and having blood tests. Both had been more positive but still nothing that I felt was definitive enough to have led us to a pregnancy. The optimist within me couldn't help but hope. I hadn't taken a pregnancy test in a year, not since my periods had disappeared and I gave up testing after the tenth negative. Before this all began. I knew I had to, if only to clear up what was going on in my body. I held my breath.

Was it? Was that a second line? I couldn't be sure. A shadow maybe, dodgy light, my imagination playing tricks on me? Was it just that I wanted to see one so desperately that I could see something that wasn't there? All of these questions swirled around in my mind at a million miles an hour. I waited for my husband to return home from work that evening.

'Do you see it?' My face crumpled, desperately wanting him to say I wasn't seeing things.

'I think so. I can't be sure though. Why don't you do another in the morning?'

Great. Like I am going to be able to sleep on this, I thought.

The next morning, I stumbled into the bathroom at 5:30am before Nico left for work, another cheapy Amazon test strip in hand. (I had decided to invest in bumper packs of both ovulation and HCG testing strips as, quite frankly, I was sick of wasting my money on them at high-street prices only to be given bad news each time. I saw it as an investment.)

There was a line. It was faint but it was there. I showed Nico again. He agreed, a faint line, but *definitely* something.

I spent the rest of the day not daring to get excited while simultaneously wanting to jump for joy. Could this be it? Was I right that this was set to work for us first time? After all of the horrible things I had read about Clomid on the internet (don't read them, by the way) – all of the '*It didn't work for me*' comments in forums – and from the few people I had managed to speak to who had had the pleasure of taking it . . .

The next morning, my little bubble of hope well and truly burst. I dragged myself into the bathroom for another early-morning test to show Nico before he left for work again. I was hoping to see that little line get darker but: nothing. There was nothing there.

Instantly I felt empty again. As if that tiny light of optimism inside me had been swiftly snuffed out.

Tears pricked at my eyes. 'It's OK. It's OK,' I heard my husband repeating over and over while rubbing my back as I sat on the edge of the bed. He had to go to work and I could tell he didn't want to leave me. I pulled the covers back over my head and went back to sleep, tears streaming down my face.

When I woke up a few hours later, I decided to test again. Goodness knows why. A glutton for punishment, perhaps? The eternal optimist, some might say. Either way, I wanted one of those little strips to give me a second opinion.

Blank again. But *how*? I held them up in the daylight, leaning up against the window, and then under the stark, bright spotlights of the bathroom. Nothing. Yet the ones from the previous day's testing were still there with their little (fading) faint lines.

I had read online about people experiencing something called a chemical pregnancy. When the egg fertilises, your body begins to produce a small amount of pregnancy hormone, which can sometimes be enough to get a positive test, but then that little embryo fails to implant into the uterine wall, making for a failed pregnancy. Most people, who weren't obsessively trying to get pregnant or watching their cycles like a hawk as I had been, probably wouldn't have even known it had happened – a later period maybe, a complete non-event in some people's worlds. I, however, had already played out the whole sorry state of affairs in my mind over and over again, blaming my barely there lining as the cause of the failure.

Failure. That word again. I didn't want to feel like one, or to feel like my body had failed us, but I couldn't help it. I remember crying and crying that day and just willing my period to show up already and put me out of this misery.

It didn't come. Another ten days passed and a panic trip to the Early Pregnancy Unit to have a scan just to check that there wasn't an ectopic pregnancy also ensued. We were due to go on our holiday in less than two weeks and I just wanted to know what on earth was going on inside me. I had done everything right this cycle, everything by the book, and still this was the outcome. When my period eventually showed up, I honestly felt relieved that I could just move on from that first experience of Clomid and give the second round a shot.

I took it again, same dosage, and a week later we were off on holiday. Finally, a warmer climate, a reason to be cheerful. I felt as though I left all of my fertility on the tarmac at Heathrow and made the conscious decision just to enjoy a week of exactly what I fancied – eating, reading books uninterrupted and sipping on a few Aperol Spritz. Bliss. Of course, not one to give up too easily, I didn't forget my Chinese herbs and continued to take them each morning and evening with the help of our hotel room kettle. Still disgusting, even on a different continent.

The week raced past. It was exactly what we had both longed for, a much-needed break and, returning home, I felt like I had managed to offload much of the weight of the previous months. It was like pressing a reset button.

Though, just in case you're wondering – that age-old piece of advice of 'Just book a holiday' and you'll be sure to get pregnant . . . yeah, that one's not true either. Not even with the help of fertility drugs, it would seem. I was, at least, learning to laugh at it all. 'Just go on holiday, that's what you need,' was advice I heard from so many people and it was infuriating. Imagine that every time we wanted to get pregnant we just told ourselves to 'relax', booked a holiday and voila! I know, I'm being facetious, as my mother would say.

So the holiday was lovely but the Clomid didn't work its magic that month either. It did give me a newly shortened 26-day cycle, though. I was gearing up to see my consultant the following week and couldn't wait to regale to her the trials and tribulations of my clomiphene adventures thus far. Not.

I wasn't really sure what to expect that day as I sat down ready for the latest 'What next?' chat. My scan showed I hadn't ovulated in the shorter cycle and that it was too early to tell in this (third) cycle whether either ovary was responding with a dominant follicle. I filled her in on cycle one and she had also heard from the Early Pregnancy Unit that I had been in to check up on things. She agreed that it could have been a chemical pregnancy but that (of course) it was impossible to diagnose. I think she could tell the glimmer of hope it had given me and that I was truly invested in my Clomid experience to date.

Because of the less-than-definitive start with these first three rounds, we agreed that if nothing happened in this cycle then the fourth to sixth cycles would be on a higher, double dose, of clomiphene. She also advised me to stop the metformin and continue with the patches as normal. It was becoming hard to keep up! If I was confused then god only knows what was going on inside me. I wouldn't have been surprised if my ovaries had opted to stay behind in Dubai on an extended break. Surely it had to be better than facing this monthly drug cocktail?

I left clutching a further prescription and agreeing I'd be back again in August. We had discussed IVF again, with the possibility that a referral would be made in September if these last rounds of Clomid didn't bring success. I didn't even know how I felt about it anymore. It seemed as though the prospect of more invasive treatment was getting ever closer to being our reality so I may as well see it as something to look forward to as opposed to something to dread. I decided to read more about it, listen to some podcasts, inform myself about what might be to come.

The next three months flew past us. Teddy's second birthday came and went. I had been certain that by this point there would have been a younger sibling at least on the horizon, but not yet. We spent it having a rainy picnic on Sandbanks beach in Dorset, a happy place where we had got engaged just five years previously. We got soaked and laughed about it. It felt like a sign, us laughing in the face of the metaphorical soaking that the last two years had given us. An absolute downpour.

June, July and into August were another two rounds of Clomid fun. The last two before seriously discussing IVF. Number of pregnancies? Zero. Number of sticks peed on? I definitely lost count. On this Clomid roller-coaster, my cycles had lasted anywhere from 26 to 48 days, so it was a minefield of sheer confusion. There were many ups and downs and many ugly tears. The whole thing had felt quite remarkable, and not in a good way. Next month we would be going into Autumn. My entire year so far had been buried under a mountain of drugs and what-ifs. I didn't know exactly what my next appointment would hold but I knew it would be the time we had *that* conversation. That the next part of the plan would be on the table. That actually, after all was said and done, after all the drugs and the herbs and the sticks that had been peed on, we were, in fact, *just going to do IVF*.

Chapter 5

Happy but Heartbroken

'CONGRATULATIONS. LOVELY NEWS. I'M SO HAPPY FOR YOU.'

It wasn't a lie, I was. Happy for them, I mean. I had just become weary of repeatedly punching out these words in a message or social media comment. I am, of course, talking about other people's pregnancy news. Happy news! Excited announcements of an impending arrival!

It's a subject we tend to skirt around within the community of people who are trying to conceive, one that I feel we don't give nearly enough airtime to. Understandably, we don't want to upset anyone, especially our closest friends or family, but at the same time, I think we owe it to ourselves, to our own sanity, to be able to acknowledge all of the emotions that those announcements of other people's pregnancies can often bring. It's not that we are not happy for them – I believe it's a natural reaction to be happy and excited for someone you love and are close to when they tell you they are expecting, even if you're struggling to get there yourself. However, I think it's also important to know that those feelings, sharing in their happiness, love and joy, can also coexist next to your own overwhelming disappointment.

When we want something so badly for ourselves and we are trying so hard to get it, it's natural that it stings a little when someone else gets there first, or gets there again. There were times when friends would announce a second, or even third pregnancy, and I would be thinking, 'I just want a chance for one. One to take home.' I didn't feel like I was asking for much, and I wasn't. As my mum would say, 'Some people make it look as easy as shelling peas.' Annoyingly, she's right. They really did. I also had to remind myself that I didn't always know the full story of what it might have taken other people to get there.

Pregnancy announcements didn't always upset me but there were a few I found more triggering than others.

And still do. Personally, I really struggle with scan pictures – I don't know why exactly. I never showed one to anyone other than my closest friends and family when we were expecting Teddy. I didn't feel like a photograph of the inside of my uterus was something I wanted to be out there for public consumption and my experiences of the last four years have only compounded that. It feels like a private place and, no matter who was currently inhabiting it, it isn't somewhere I wanted scrolled past or 'liked' through the window of social media. I suppose I also didn't like the thought of the world at large seeing our baby before we had had the opportunity to meet him or her for ourselves. That sounds crazy, I know – it's just a picture, and not a very good one at that!

Then, after Teddy died, I began to dislike scan pictures even more. Facebook seemed awash with them on a regular basis so I decided, as a method of self-preservation during a particularly tough time, it would be a better idea to delete the app from my phone altogether. This was the sort of step I felt I had to take in order to protect my own heart. It wasn't that I wasn't overjoyed that someone I had gone to school with over 15 years ago – and hadn't seen for the entirety of that 15 years – was expecting (again), it was just that I needed to shelter myself from it, for now.

I got to a point with Instagram where the mute button on people's stories and posts became my best friend. A handy ally I could call upon when I needed some help. Pregnancy and birth announcements were plentiful. There were days I could handle them and days when I couldn't. Some announcements came after long struggles and were sensitively made, not wanting to upset others even in their own happiest moment. These I delighted in and they rarely made me cry anything other than genuinely happy tears. Others stung a little more than I'd care to freely admit, even from friends. Clutching bumps, scans, pegboards of 'Coming October 2018 . . .' *How could they be so sure*, I thought. With just a 12-week scan in the bag there's still a 20-week anomaly scan to get through. How could anyone, ever, be so sure that it was all going to be OK?

I had to accept that those feelings were created from my own experiences after my own worst fears had been realised in May 2016. That this was what kept me from being able to enjoy that sheer joy, naivety or 'knowing' everything was going to be OK, ever again. I think now that a lot of what ran through me was actually envy – I wished I could be so certain that I would bring a healthy baby home. To be so certain that I even put a date on it.

I didn't know whether those posts made me sad for myself or whether I was just consumed with fear for them that something might go wrong; either way, they never felt comfortable. The onslaught of bump-clutching photos and early nursery prep that then followed was usually enough to have me hitting the mute button within weeks. Most of these kinds of announcements weren't from real-life friends but from people I had chosen to follow on my social media. I was, of course, free to unfollow them at any time and sometimes I did. There were other times when I found myself in situations where I knew I would risk upsetting that person if I took those actions, even though their posts were upsetting and triggering me more than they could possibly ever understand. That was when mute was my only friend.

After Teddy died, I had made a close-knit group of friends with some other 'loss mums', as we thought of ourselves. We had met online and bonded over dark humour, a love of baking and a passion for talking openly and honestly about our babies. We called ourselves the Warrior Women and set up a little WhatsApp chat for daily banter and camaraderie at our darkest times. That was summer 2016, now over two years ago, and I was also the only one of the seven of us who was yet to become a mum again.

At first, I had felt certain that we would all get our rainbows within months of one another. A rainbow baby is a baby born after loss; miscarriage, stillbirth, neonatal death. The rainbow after the storm, I suppose. If the universe had taken away from us all, then surely it was set to give back in a timely fashion too? The first flurry of rainbows arrived during April, May and June 2017, with another in May the following year and one set to arrive in September 2018. All had brought me so much joy for each of those girls I was now lucky enough to call my friend, and each one had helped to bolster my hope that it might happen again for us, too. But with three of those rainbows already toddling and mine nowhere to be seen, I couldn't help my feelings of elation for everyone else being coupled with my own hopelessness, overshadowing everything.

All of the girls were so loving, so supportive and so understanding, whether I did or didn't want to talk about our current situation. I had always honestly shared with them my ups and downs of the many drugs I had tried and the prospect of IVF that lay ahead for us. They did their very best to keep my spirits up and my hopes high but I was beginning to believe that another baby might not be in my future. Surely law of averages and statistics state that not all seven of us could get a healthy take-home baby after all of this? There had to be winners and losers, the lucky and the unlucky, and I feared I was the latter.

I'm well aware that having a rainbow baby after loss isn't ever the 'happy ending' society might like us to believe it will be. Being able to parent a living child doesn't simply eradicate all that has come before it. We still bear the pain, every day; we still look at that living child and wonder whether he or she is some reflection or image of who or what that sibling might have been. There is still the yearning to hold that other child, just once more, or get to parent both of them at the same time. I wasn't under the illusion that these women were miraculously 'cured' of their grief, or that having another child and parenting after loss hadn't added even more layers and complexities to an already complicated journey. But I was aching to hold my own living baby and starting to wonder whether that prospect might be slipping away from me.

Announcements came and went, and I tried reframing these emotions each time in a different way to make myself feel less guilty for experiencing them. It's hard to admit aloud to anyone that someone else's happiness is making you feel sad, no matter what your situation. I didn't want anyone to think I was wallowing and I wasn't sure if I should share my true feelings with anyone other than my husband for fear of being seen as jealous or cruel. How do you say to a friend, 'I'm really happy for you, but I'm just sad it's not me,' without completely taking away from their happy announcement?

So I became a master of the 'Congratulations!' poker face. Genuinely sharing in their happiness for the time that I had to sit it out face-to-face and then usually resorting to desperate sobs once alone again in the sanctuary of my home/car/out on a walk. Sometimes I would find myself driving or walking alone and suddenly being aware of the tears that were streaming down my cheeks as I had thought too much about someone else's happy news, or pondered the prospect of yet more friends telling me they were expecting. Like some kind of strange subconscious chemical reaction happening in my body again and again, trying to release the pain and pressure of the past two years.

I began to feel like I had a new heightened sense of awareness, ready to sniff out any potential pregnancy announcement when so much as a hint of suspicion became apparent. Friend gone quiet on me? Must be pregnant. Cancelled plans? Yep, she's expecting. I felt if I could pre-empt it before being served the final blow by text or phone call, if I could at least see it coming, then I could reassure myself as the news was delivered that, *Well, you knew she was anyway*. That, somehow, that would make it better. Right? The truth is that this tactic didn't work at all. It just made me neurotically suspicious of anyone who dared to be of child-bearing age. I really didn't want to be that person.

On one occasion when a friend told me she was pregnant again, I was just getting out of the car to go to an acupuncture appointment (and to pick up some more of those delightful herbs!). I glanced at my phone before I walked into the waiting room. The tone of her message was apologetic. She wanted to tell me before she let any of our other friends know that she was pregnant with their third. She said that she hadn't had her 12-week scan just yet but she had seen me a few weeks previously and the weight of the guilt she had been feeling over me was already eating away at her. She explained that she couldn't wait any longer to tell me because she needed me to know in case I chose to distance myself from her. She said she would understand

and that, although she had wanted this pregnancy, she also knew how much I wanted that for myself.

I stopped dead on the pavement, frozen to the ground. At first, I felt that familiar rise of panic in my chest, the tears stinging at the back of my eyes, threatening to fall down my cheeks at any given moment. I knew there was no one around me who I was afraid of being embarrassed in front of. No one to see what I was crying about, or to judge me for being apparently sad at someone else's happiness. There was nothing to stop me from bursting into tears right there and then if I felt like it. This time, though, I didn't.

Something in her message hit me right in the face. Her words, her empathy for my situation and my feelings, even though I knew she'd never experienced pregnancy loss or fertility challenges herself. She was openly telling me that she felt guilty, that she had wished this for me as much as she had ever wished if for herself. Even further, that she'd understand if it was so painful for me that I couldn't see her or didn't feel I could congratulate her. She was the first friend who had openly acknowledged those feelings of mine, who truly seemed to empathise with what it might be like to be on the receiving end of someone else's happy news. She had gone so far as to put herself in my shoes, to consider how and when she might tell me. Then she'd left the door open for me to close it in her face if I felt I needed to for my own self-preservation.

I didn't reply immediately, I let her words sit with me and I walked into my appointment. As I lay there with my eyes closed and those needles tingling in my skin I re-read her text in my mind over and over, putting myself in her shoes and then back into mine, just as she must have done in the build-up to sending that message. I swung in and out of my own feelings of disappointment and grief and back over to her feeling of guilt.

When I came out of the appointment, feeling a million times lighter and with a much clearer head, I pulled my phone from my bag and began to type, writing, deleting and re-writing as I walked. With my reply finally clear in my mind, I pressed send. I told her I didn't want her to worry about me. That pretty much every woman I knew had fallen pregnant by this point. I reassured her that I was really and truly happy for her, and I meant that. I never wanted her to feel guilty, I never wanted any of my friends to feel that way, and my heart ached a little that I might have started to make other people feel like that. She was the first person who made me acknowledge those feelings properly and learn to sit with them.

It's so easy to look at someone else's circumstances and only see part of the picture, the part you want to see, that allows you to indulge in those feelings of jealousy or resentment. I had to try to keep focusing on my own journey, not theirs. Looking at someone else's path and wanting to make it your own doesn't get you anywhere; looking at yours and realising what you can do to get where you want to be, can. I didn't want to be an expert in anyone else's fertility, or know how or why they had fallen pregnant, I wanted to know what I could do to help myself get there.

It was just like Emma had said to me in that consultation a year previously: 'Each time you are struggling, losing focus, feeling lost, I want you to remind yourself and ask yourself – why do you want another baby?' The focus was always on the word 'you' and it had taken me a year to see that. It wasn't about anyone else, or their path, it was about me. Looking at someone else's wouldn't change where mine was heading, no matter how much I longed for their happy news to become mine. I certainly shouldn't punish people or push them away, but just let them know, gently, why that news might take a little longer for me to digest. It wasn't that I wasn't happy, I was just a little bit heartbroken, and that's OK.

Chapter 6

Ding, Ding! Round One

I COULDN'T BELIEVE THAT WE WERE ACTUALLY SITTING HERE. It was mid-August and after a meeting with my consultant earlier that month that confirmed what we had all suspected, that my Clomid and hormone cocktail had unsuccessfully run its course, we were onto the next step. IVF.

The referral for the initial steps had happened really quickly. First we had to attend an appointment to fill in paperwork with a registrar. So we found ourselves sat at a different hospital, waiting for our turn to step into the little room behind the door in front of us. The door opened and a smiling face greeted us. She was an older lady who explained she worked directly for the

IVF consultant on 'eligibility of new referrals'. As we were ushered in and tentatively took our seats on the opposite side of the room to her, that word rang so loudly in my mind.

Eligibility.

Hang on. Was this not a given then? What further criteria could there possibly be to fulfil in order to be 'eligible'? It was almost four years since we had begun trying for a baby and way over two since Teddy had died and we had begun 'trying again'. My mind stopped dead when I began to consider that we might not fall into the eligible category.

Two clipboards were duly handed to each of us, both stacked with forms to be filled out. They included all of the usual things: name, medical history, medication, height, weight, number of children . . . That was always the question I stumbled upon. I looked up from her and said, 'This part . . .'

'Yes?' she replied, smiling again.

'Well, we have a son, but he, he . . .' My words trailed off as I fell into silence and the lump in my throat took hold.

'He died when he was a baby. Not long after he was born.' Thank goodness Nico could find the words.

'Ah yes, I did see that information in your referral notes. I'm so sorry, I should have said. It's really referring to number of *living* children. So just put none in that box.'

Just like that, it was as if he never existed. I was shaking. I didn't know if it was fear or upset. Obviously, we had to put '0' in that box or I imagine our eligibility for an NHS-funded round of IVF would have been approximately zero. Still, it pained me to see it in black and white as my answer.

The forms seemed to take an age to complete, repeating the same information over and over. Hospital numbers, signatures – some papers we both had to sign and some were just for us as individuals. It was such a thorough process and no stone was left unturned. All the while, the registrar explained to us what the next steps of the process might look like. She said that all the paperwork went to their main office where each couple's case would go in front of a panel who took all of the relevant information into consideration before agreeing to funding or not. If successful, the go-ahead would then be given to the IVF wing at the local private IVF hospital that they partnered with. Any treatment would then proceed from there with the same IVF/fertility consultant who worked between both hospitals. We would have an initial meeting with them, a treatment plan would be put in place and any cycle of treatment could then proceed (our health and my cycle timings permitting). Perhaps even this side of Christmas, with a little good luck and a prevailing wind behind us?

It seemed like utter madness to be already leaping ahead four months to Christmas when we were barely nearing the end of the summer, but when you have spent the entirety of your year so far wishing away the months from cycle to cycle, what's another four if it brings some good news?

Before we left, I was measured and weighed (something I had become used to in previous pregnancies, so it made me feel a little less like cattle going up for auction now). We were also told that we would need to go for blood tests right there and then to test our blood types and to check for certain diseases such as hepatitis, HIV and others.

We said goodbye to the kind registrar and made our way along the hospital corridors to haematology, where we took our waiting-room tickets from the little machine on the wall and patiently waited for our numbers to be called out. I remember watching my husband as he turned his ticket over and over between his fingertips and nervously tapped his feet together on the floor. In that moment it struck me: this was the first time in any of our treatment, in this entire journey so far, that *he* was also going to be subject to the poking and prodding, the questions and tests. Up until this point he had sat on the sidelines as a helpless bystander, cheering me on, rubbing my back and telling me it was going to be OK. He had suddenly become, very much, a part of this process; a cog in the fertility machine that was going to propel us to our destination. This was on both of us now.

Another thing that had been arranged for the following week was a sperm sample. Again, another thing that he'd *have* to be involved in – taking a starring role, in fact. It made perfect sense that if all corners of my reproductive system were going to be investigated, his should, at the very least, come under a little scrutiny too. The process was run like a military operation with a time-window in which the sample pot had to be collected and returned to the hospital. He would then receive the results via post and then we eventually met with the IVF consultant. Part of me felt a glimmer of smugness that finally it wasn't just me being tested for something. Of course, the other half of me was petrified that this would prove to be a further stumbling block, something else that we hadn't been expecting. They were looking at sperm count and morphology – basically, were the numbers good and did they all look to be in working order? After much laughing about the process as a whole, the deed was done, sample dropped off and we waited. Again.

September saw us take a break in our favourite place, Cornwall. It was where we always escaped to when things got too much; the place we had retreated to the very week after Teddy had died. This break was a little different though, as my first book had finally been published that week. I had needed a break from the whirlwind that had been the build-up to its release and we both needed some time off from all things fertility-based. Our blood tests and the sperm sample had all come back clear/healthy/normal. My husband's sperm count was high, leading to many an inappropriate joke about super-sperm and such like.

Obviously, I was relieved, we both were, but at the same time that weight of responsibility, of blame, even, crept back onto my shoulders, pressing down with the thought that it would be my fault if we couldn't have more children. However, I was taking a break from the *delicious* Chinese herbs and hadn't been on any kind of hormone or drug for a good four weeks now and I was feeling alive again. Everything was finally making its way out of my system. Each blustery beach walk we went on I felt the sluggishness and mind-fog of the last 14 months slowing washing away. Everything felt better, I had more energy and my skin was beginning to look less like decomposing flesh and more like *me* again. I knew this wouldn't be a permanent fixture, that we were staring straight down the barrel of something much bigger, but I wanted to relish in these little life-wins for as long as we were here. It was a welcome break from it all, for my body and mind.

The IVF referral was never far from our minds, though. I checked my phone calendar week by week, counting down the days from the moment we had stepped out of that last appointment. She had said up to six weeks and we were fast approaching five. I was certain there would be a letter waiting for us on the doormat upon our return from Cornwall. But there was not.

After a beautiful break, I immediately felt catapulted back into that vortex of waiting and worrying, knowing that the decision would have likely been made and it was entirely out of our control. The following week came and I couldn't wait any longer. I called the department at the hospital where our referral appointment had been to ask if there was any progress. The lady I spoke to sounded perplexed as to why we hadn't heard anything and was helpful enough to give me the name and contact number of the person who dealt with application eligibility. After a morning of calling, leaving messages and waiting, I finally got a call back from the department I had been trying to reach.

'I'm really sorry,' he said. 'There seems to have been some confusion with your application. Your paperwork never made it to us so the process hasn't actually started.'

I felt so crestfallen. Six weeks of waiting, for what? We were back to the bottom of the pile, the back of the queue, when I had been so certain this wait was nearly over. I cried on the phone as his words 'I'm so sorry, I don't know what to say' echoed in my ears.

Before I hung up the phone I asked him if he could email me the details of what had happened. He agreed. I'd say he definitely recognised the sound of a desperate woman when he heard one.

I called my husband, my words barely coherent on the telephone: 'It's fucked. It's not happening.'

More than a little dramatic at this point, I realise that now, but it felt like my world had come crashing down that day. More endless waiting. His voice was the calming and reassuring tonic that I needed. He simply said, 'Well, why don't you forward that email covering what's happened on to our consultant and see if she can help us?'

He was right. Of course, she would at least be able to ask the question as to what had gone wrong. I emailed her secretary and my GP, as both had been so helpful and so instrumental in getting us this far. I was certain they'd want to know if the wheels had come off in any part of the process. Both got back to me that same day and had contacted the applications office to request that our eligibility decision be fast-tracked given the wait we had already endured. We had so many people in our corner, fighting for us, *with* us, I couldn't believe it. I knew this whole process had the potential of swallowing us both whole, making us lose our minds and ourselves along the way, it felt so reassuring to know that we had so much support around us.

Their persistence paid off and I received an email later that week to say that our application had been fast-tracked, considered and approved. I actually screamed with excitement. I never imagined I could have felt so elated at the prospect of a round of IVF, but I did!

Because even a single round of IVF might mean a baby, and that was all we wanted.

It was autumn by the time we were finally sitting in front of the IVF consultant at the hospital. Our first consultation was a meeting to go over what would be the best treatment plan for us. We were both nervous, unsure of what it would entail. Terrified, we walked into the IVF wing of the hospital and up the stairs to the reception desk. As I looked up at the walls of the stairwell and corridors, I saw gallery frames staring back at me all filled with photo upon photo of newborn, bouncing babies. Gummy smiles and wide eyes; twins upon twins. Something swelled up inside me. I think it was hope.

Yes, hope.

The consultant was everything I had hoped he would be. He was understanding, listened to us, had taken the time to read about Teddy and wanted to let us know how sorry he was that we were now facing these challenges too. He explained to us, based on all of our test results and my obstetric history, what his preferred treatment plan for IVF would be. It was a short, or flare, protocol, as it is sometimes called, involving two weeks of stimulation injections, followed by a trigger to release any eggs, then an egg retrieval procedure and then, all being well, an embryo transfer at day five if we had a healthy embryo that made it that far. He was so knowledgeable, he almost made it sound simple.

We would need to wait until I had had my next period, followed by a pelvic assessment scan (I feared that would almost certainly be another dalliance with the dildo wand) and then we would have our 'booking appointment' with the nurses to go over our treatment plan in detail and check off every form that had been filled in along the way. Following all of that, treatment could go ahead. We would certainly be in by Christmas.

Pregnant by Christmas, even? My nerves melted away; inside I was jumping for joy. I think if it had been socially acceptable, I would have done so right there and then in his office.

My scan (a dildo-wand-extravaganza indeed) followed a couple of weeks later, with our booking appointment a few days after that. The scan turned out to be a blink-and-you'll-miss-it kind of affair, whereas we were told to prepare for the booking appointment to last two hours. I couldn't believe that there could actually be any more forms to fill in. Yet, there were. Check boxes and signatures a plenty. I understood why, of course – there were serious questions to be considered here, things I had never even contemplated. Like, for example, would my husband give me permission to use any embryos we had in the event of him dying before our transfer date? Blimey. Heavy stuff. I could only assume these questions had become part of the process because these situations had actually arisen. We ticked and ticked and signed our lives away until it felt like the last of the paperwork was finally complete.

We were asked about the number of embryos that were to be put 'back in', as it were. The consultant's recommendation was one (based on my age of 33 and my previous obstetric history) and we decided to tick the 'up to two' box if the situation were to arise that we had two less-than-grade-A embryos left to choose from. This meant both would be transferred in the hope that one successful single pregnancy would be achieved, so not an effort to achieve a potential twin pregnancy. This seemed like a sensible option to take if it were there.

The last part of the appointment was to go through the drugs I would take and what each would do. The nurse explained how the injections were to be administered and what each medication would do. The first few days of injections were a stimulation drug; this was to get those ovaries growing some follicles. After that, a second injection would be added into the mix; this one was to prevent my body from actually releasing any eggs from those follicles, to basically hold on to everything until the time was right for egg retrieval. The injections were to be done every evening, between 6pm and 8pm, with the nurse's advice being that once I had picked a time to try and always do the injection within a 30-minute window either side of that time. During these two weeks of injections, I would be coming into the clinic every two to three days for progress scans to track the follicles and count how many and how big they were, so that the optimum day for egg retrieval could be ascertained. Once egg retrieval had been arranged, the last appointment before that would see me leave with a trigger injection to administer before the big day. Exciting stuff. A trigger is the final injection of the round; a drug designed to encourage all of those follicles you've been cultivating during treatment to finally release those eggs ready for collection.

After all of this had been explained and we had watched the nurse draw medication up into syringes from bottles multiple times as she walked through each step, she asked if we had any questions or concerns. My husband responded with a quick no, while I replied nervously, 'I've never given myself an injection before.'

Truth being that I was more than a little worried I was going to fuck this up totally at one point or another.

'Would you like to try a practice run now?' she asked, cheerily proffering a syringe in my direction.

Oh *shit*. How did I know she was going to ask that? I wish I had, just for once, kept my mouth shut. My fear was evidently palpable in the room at this point as she continued in an encouraging manner: 'You won't feel it, they are tiny needles, similar to diabetic needles. I'll talk you through it as you go.'

Her kindness and confidence must have bolstered me at this point because the next thing I knew I was squeezing tightly onto the fleshiest part of my tummy as I plunged a practice-run needle right into it.

'There!' she said triumphantly. 'That was easy, wasn't it?'

She was right. Surprisingly easy, actually. My husband, who up until this point had been sitting there agreeing with the nurse and telling me how it wouldn't hurt and how I needn't be scared, suddenly got the shock of his life as she turned to him and said, 'Right then. Your turn.'

The look on his face was a picture. I was hooting with laughter.

'Weren't expecting that, were you?' I chuckled. 'Telling me how easy it is . . .'

I couldn't be sure if she was joking or not but she then proceeded to explain that lots of partners like to try it out too so that they can see what it's like, and also if they are going to be helping out with injections. Thankfully for this partner-in-crime, I let him off that day as I could see on his face that the thought petrified him . . . ha!

We left with a treatment schedule of potential dates mapped out in front of us. If everything went to plan, and my period played ball, we would be starting drugs before the end of November and an embryo transfer would be on the cards by the end of the first week of December. By some small miracle, my period did (for once) become a reliable force and I was back in the clinic by 21st November. Before I knew it, I was back out of the door again with my next bag of goodies and treatment plan in hand. I actually felt excited! We had told few people we were starting as I didn't want to add any extra pressure into the mix. I let my parents and a couple of friends know what was happening, although I almost immediately regretted telling any friends as I quickly learned that even that pressure was too much for me. I know that some people would find the support of other people knowing a huge comfort but I found it almost unbearable. The 'How's it going?', 'How are you feeling?' questions rolled in and, even from just a few people, it set my head spinning. The reality of potentially having to tell people it hadn't worked began to set in. I tried my best to give away as little detail as possible.

The injections were easy enough and I found myself quickly getting into a rhythm with them. I set an alarm on my phone every evening so that I wouldn't forget. I was still attending my acupuncture appointments and was trying to practise a slow yoga flow every day. I was walking every day too, making sure I took time away from my laptop screen and the stresses of technology. All of the book events and promotions were over for now, which meant I could use this time fully to re-focus, re-frame and rest. There was no expectation of me other than for my body to respond well to these drugs, so that's all I was trying to help it do. The only real side effects I began to feel were tiredness and an extreme thirst, I think because you're forcing your body to do something with such force and so quickly. It must have been exhausting for those little ovaries, who were usually only expected to pop out one decent-sized follicle a month. Now they were being pumped full of drugs to make them produce ten, perhaps even twenty times that.

It was hard to think about what was going on inside there but I took some guidance from one of Emma's books and tried to visualise it each day as I was out on my walks, envisioning those little follicles growing big and strong. I know it sounds crazy but I would walk along in the woods, repeating affirmations to myself in an attempt to get things going. *I am healthy, I am fertile, and my body is ready to have another baby* on repeat. As you know by now, I really was willing to try anything.

It wasn't long before my first scan to check how my follicles were fairing came around. I was a week into my new medication routine, my belly was already beginning to resemble a slightly battered pin cushion, but I felt positive that things were working. The waiting corridor for scans was always filled with nervous-looking women, most scrolling phones or tapping their feet as they looked nervously at the floor. No one ever really chatted, not that I saw. It seemed strange, as we were all in this wondrously shitty boat together, all clinging to the liferaft of assisted fertility to help our dreams come true, but it was as if we were all holding our breath before we stepped into that room. We were all just trying to survive the next few minutes. No one was here for friendly chit-chat or banter and so it was that only nervous smiles and knowing faces were exchanged.

My scan went well. The stimulation drugs were working; those little follicles were tracking in the right direction. She checked the number and size and said I would be due back for a repeat scan in a few days. My next stop was to see the nurse, who showed me how the follicles were tracking on a little graph. She explained that during each progress scan we needed to see those little crosses going on an upward trajectory and once they reached the right size we would be arranging egg retrieval. She asked me how I was feeling and how the injections were going. I remember smiling and nodding a lot and just wanting to press fast forward on the next week to see where this took us. I practically ran down to the pharmacy to pick up my next few days' of medication, and that was that. I felt like I was nailing this whole process. I didn't feel sick, wasn't overly bloated and didn't seem to be experiencing any of the nastier side effects I had read about on various forums, or been warned about in previous appointments. I wasn't a fan of forums, as I felt that sometimes they could be a minefield of opinions as opposed to facts, and they tended to make me worry more than bring reassurance. That said, I do think they bring a wonderful sense of community and support and provide a safe place of understanding for women going through fertility struggles.

Every appointment was scheduled the same: scan, see nurse, pick up prescription and go. It was like a well-oiled baby-making machine, where couples lined the corridors waiting for their fate to be decided. My next appointment was less straightforward than the last, though, with my follicle growth having slowed down somewhat and lots of smaller follicles appearing to be waiting in the wings. The upward trajectory of those little crosses seemed to be flattening but my nurse that day didn't panic. After a quick chat with the consultant, it was decided to increase my stimulation dose for the next few days before the next scan, which would help to give those little follicles a welcome boost (fingers crossed). As the nurse didn't seem too worried, I tried not to be either. I did feel a little deflated though. This felt like the first bump in the road. Why were my ovaries seemingly so pedantic about every bloody thing I requested of them? She advised me to rest, drink plenty of water and keep doing what I had been doing before my next scan. So that's what I did. I would spend the weekend doing absolutely nothing; I wanted to give my body the best chance to do this.

The weekend seemed to go on for an eternity. All I wanted to know was what was happening in there. I had been on stimulation drugs for 12 days now. Originally my egg retrieval had been pencilled in for early that week but it looked as though that would be pushed back now. It was already the first week of December – the waiting and the lead up to all of this had made the months fly by. It was the week of my husband's birthday and I so wanted it to be a week that finally brought us some good fortune. I was praying for a Christmas miracle.

As the nurse scanned over my ovaries, the room felt eerily quiet, other than the usually process of her calling out numbers as I scrawled down each one on a piece of paper. I think the clinic used this as a method of getting you involved in the process but also to aid the visualisation for patients of what was going on in there.

'Twelve, twelve, fourteen, sixteen . . .' she continued.

I knew these numbers were still small – she was talking in millimetres. I counted only one, maybe two, on my list of numbers in front of me that would be anywhere near big enough for them to consider egg retrieval. I didn't speak much. Instead I listened to the tone of her voice and watched her manner as she spoke. I knew it wasn't the best news. As I followed the nurse into the next room a few minutes later my eyes locked on the chart in her hands.

'Really, to proceed to egg retrieval with the confidence that we would harvest enough mature eggs to achieve successful fertilisation, we would be looking for a number of three to five decent-sized follicles at the very least.'

'How many do I have?' I asked without skipping a beat.

'You have one.'

One. *One* fucking follicle. Two weeks of injections and one measly follicle. I honestly didn't know whether to laugh or cry. A chemical reaction in my body was far stronger and it chose the latter. She immediately handed me a box of tissues.

'Does this happen often?' I questioned.

'Not all that often but it does happen. At this point we would cancel this treatment round and you can opt to have a trigger injection to take home to help your body release the egg from that follicle. Then you are free to try naturally this month.'

All of this and we were back to relying on Mother Nature being kind to us. I couldn't quite believe it.

'OK, well, we might as well try that. What next?'

'We can get a review appointment booked for you in the New Year to discuss this treatment plan and how we could improve things for next time. Then you could look to start again in the New Year, if you felt ready?'

So, that was that. Round one, over before it had really started. What had it all been for? What had we learned from this?

I didn't know. All I knew was that I couldn't wait to get out of there that day and I couldn't wait for this year of waiting for nothing to be over.

Chapter 7

Christmas is Cancelled

THE CAR JOURNEY HOME WAS A BLUR. I don't recall the drive other than blubbing as I listened to my husband try to reassure me through the car phone speakers. I had called him straight away, of course, to tell him that my ovaries had stuck two fingers up at us once more and that Christmas was cancelled. (Third year running. Rather impressive.) He asked me if I needed him to come home. I didn't see that there was anything either of us could do or say to make this better, so I encouraged him to stay put. I didn't want my dark cloud to rain over him too.

When I returned home my mum was the next person to pick up a sob-filled phone call (I was just a spreader of joy today!). Like Nico, she tried her best to comfort me and I knew she truly empathised with how this must have felt for us. I felt as though my body had let us down, that *I* had let us down, again. The weight of that burden was becoming so much to carry. It didn't seem to matter how much I tried, how I changed my life, did all of the right things or ate like a goddess of nutrition. No matter how hard I *wished* for good news, this could still be the outcome.

It was the beginning of the festive season and my social media feed was overflowing with Pinterest-perfect photos of families in front of their Christmas trees, at Christmas tree farms, visiting Father Christmas – all happy, smiling faces staring back at me. I had to take a few days off from it all to take stock of the situation before I threw my phone out of a moving vehicle. That aching feeling swirled in the pit of my stomach again and I wanted to switch it off, to numb myself to the emotions that soared when I saw happy families and bouncing babies. Was it jealousy? Or was it just a deep sadness for the things that I knew we were missing out on with Teddy and the things we had yet to experience with another child? Teddy should have been two and a half by now. Would I have got us matching pyjamas? Hell yes. December was already such a strange time for us and I had given up on trying to keep hold of any kind of feeling of control during the festivities. I had accepted that things would always be different, difficult, that little bit sadder for us. No matter what changed, even if we had more children in years to come, Teddy would *always* be missing at Christmas.

The first week following the 'bad news' appointment went past in a flash. The trigger shot was administered and I gave up any glimmer of hope before that bad boy even left the syringe. Trying for a baby wasn't on our minds now; we were in survival mode for the next few weeks. We celebrated Nico's birthday with friends, the first time I remember laughing – properly belly laughing – in a long time. A glass of wine in hand, I knocked it back and enjoyed the feeling of freedom for a while.

In a strange way, I think we both also felt a tiny sense of relief. That we had tried IVF for the first time and it hadn't been as bad as we had anticipated. That I could, in fact, administer my own injections and easily hide it from the world. That we wouldn't have to hide an early pregnancy over Christmas while we both festered in yet more worry about what it might bring. We could come clean with the rest of our family and friends that we had tried treatment and it had ended in a right royal clusterfuck before it had really got off the ground. These were tiny wins but I think we used them as a way to comfort ourselves at a time when wins were impossibly thin on the ground.

Days away from Christmas, my period arrived. Oh, the festive joy that swelled through every fibre of my being! Strangely, it actually felt like a relief, a huge release from it all, as well as it bringing the knowledge that we were on 'day one' again. A clean slate. A new start line. It also meant that I could call the clinic to give them this joyous news and I would be able to book in for our review appointment, which also meant a 'What next?' plan with our consultant. Because we had ended our cycle before egg retrieval and had no embryos to show for our efforts, we decided it would be wasteful to use that up as one of our funded cycles. So we were able to pay for the drugs and scans up to that point and start with a new, fresh, funded cycle when we were ready. It wasn't something we could really afford at the time, but we couldn't bear the thought of losing the funded cycle to something that was so incomplete; it felt too much of a waste.

When I called the clinic, I was surprised to hear that our consultant had already approved us to begin our next round, when we were ready and if we so wished. It would be changed to a long treatment protocol, meaning that I was on day two of our treatment cycle already and we were, technically, in this next round. The nurse explained that drugs would start on day 21 this time but that we wouldn't be going straight into stimulation as before. With this method, the first two weeks would include a down-regulation period by injecting a drug called buserelin. Down-regulating, as it was referred to, was a process of switching everything off to quieten the ovaries (I thought those guys were already pretty bloody quiet to be honest. Any quieter and they'd be mute!). After those two weeks, and having had a period in that time, I would have a baseline scan to make sure everything was ready to go. Then came the next part: back onto the stimulation injections again, firing up those ovaries and kick-starting them into producing some follicles. These injections would be coupled with the continuation of buserelin, which would play the part of keeping everything under control and stop the body from actually ovulating.

It was like a fine art, keeping everything perfectly balanced so as to get my body in a place where it behaved exactly as we wanted it to. Too little and we would have a repeat of last time; too much and they risked over-stimulating my already polycystic-looking ovaries. This was going to be a learning process and they couldn't tell me which way it would go. They promised they would keep a close eye on proceedings and I trusted them implicitly. Although our clinic had effectively been chosen for us, I knew they were one of the best in our area and we were incredibly fortunate to be having treatment there. I had spent lots of time reading up on their website and on other places online about their fresh and frozen cycle success rates and their live-birth rates, and studying charts based on age to try to gauge our chances of success with them. It all looked really positive. I was convinced that the last cycle had been a blip. The wrong choice for us, a case of having chosen short over long protocol and that this change would make all of the difference to our outcome.

Our day 21 appointment was made for just a few days after New Year. Just like that, my new-found freedom to indulge in a glass of wine was over before it had started! Ah well, it was a good ten days while it lasted! I had to laugh – only we could manage to get such a short-lived break from it all.

Obviously, we didn't *have* to start again so soon but after a quick discussion we both agreed that it felt the right thing to do. We had been so prepared for this process, so geared-up to see it through, and I think we both felt a bit short-changed that we hadn't even managed to get to the finish line on the first attempt, no matter if that had resulted in a pregnancy or not. We needed that completion, that closure, of a full, un-interrupted round of treatment. So it only felt right to jump back in head-first.

I also thought January would be the perfect time for treatment. No one is drinking, no one is going out (not that our social lives had been particularly wild in recent years), so it meant we could get through those weeks of treatment without too many questions or invites to dodge. It felt like the perfect crime! It also meant that Christmas, for me at least, would need to be a time that I continued to eat well, look after myself and try (desperately try) not to stress about things to come. I closed my laptop on 20th December and de-cided to give myself a two-week break from writing, from emails, from any kind of correspondence that clouded my mind. It sounds clichéd, but with Christ-mas already feeling so heavy, I just wanted to enjoy cosy log fires, hot chocolate, cheesy Christmas movies and the odd walk in the crisp December air. Simple things that would help keep that inevitable wave of grief under control and allow me to prepare for the weeks ahead.

Christmas was actually lovely. Sometimes I think when you prepare yourself for the worst, it turns out the build-up is worse than the actual day itself. We saw family, we laughed, we ate and we forgot all about the worries of the past year. Yes, Teddy was missing from the table, but I felt him there, I always did. His presence spurring us on, encouraging us to persevere when things felt tough. It was difficult watching our nieces and nephew opening their presents on Boxing Day, laughing and playing together, knowing that Teddy should have been there right in amongst the chaos. I wondered what his favourite toy would have been to open, or whether he would have insisted on 'Baby Shark' being blasted on repeat as the others did?

The bit-in-between went by in a flash and before we knew it, it was New Year's Eve. Staring down the barrel of 2019, open-ended and promising in our eyes. We chose, for the first time in a few years, to celebrate with friends. Just a small party at their house but it felt so good to be celebrating. I couldn't be sure if I was excited for the year ahead and all that it might bring us or just glad to see the back of the last year. I felt like I had been on every kind of drug and had tried my hand at every kind of alternative therapy. Goodness knows how many hospital appointments I had been to or how many needles had been stuck into my body (treatment/acupuncture, take your pick). It felt like it had been utter madness, something I hadn't ever imagined we would experience, and yet here we were, set to ride that unknown wave again.

So much good had come out of 2018 as well. Nico and his friends had cycled across France and raised over £30,000 for the NICU charity who cared for Teddy. I had written a bloody book for goodness sake, all about our son and all that we had experienced in losing him. Neither thing I had ever imagined was possible, and yet it had happened. There were so many reasons to smile, yet it was still laced with a bitter sweetness of what it had all been for. I watched as friends danced and laughed, as my husband looked happier than I had seen him in months. Were we closing the door on sadness and opening one to a year of only happy things instead? As we raised our glasses to cheers, and the clocks chimed midnight, I couldn't help but wonder and held my breath once more.

Chapter 8

Let's Go Round Again

IT WAS THE FIRST WEEK OF JANUARY, A COLD AND GREY MORNING, WHEN I FOUND MYSELF WALKING BACK INTO THE IVF CLINIC. The now familiar walk up the stairs with a thousand babies staring back at me, the smiling face of the receptionist and being back in the waiting room, nervously tapping my feet together and rubbing my hands to warm up.

That was my first appointment of many. I didn't feel as nervous this time as it felt as though I knew the drill. Although it was set to be a different protocol and different drugs, it all felt strangely familiar now, comfortable even. I even had a favourite chair in the waiting area as it meant I could make the most of people-watching as I waited. I would find myself watching people as they were ushered in and out of rooms, wondering what their story was. How long had this process been going on for them? Did they have children already? Had they suffered a loss, like us? All of these unanswered questions remained as nothing more than wandering thoughts because, as we know, this wasn't the place for chit-chat or questions.

My appointment was straightforward enough – drugs explained and injection demos repeated. We discussed buserelin and exactly how it works. The way it was explained to me was that it switches everything off, just shuts it down. Meaning no ovulation, no thickening of the lining, nothing. They likened it to the menopause – a fake menopause, if you like. As with the menopause, there could likely be side effects. Hot flushes, bloating, headaches, mood swings. What a rollercoaster ride to look forward to! Undeterred, I listened intently, made my next appointment for two weeks' time (when I would have what was called a baseline scan to see if this drug has done its thing) and then made my way down to the pharmacy. I left, once more, clutching a paper bag of drugs and needles and hoping for the best this time.

I called Nico. 'You didn't miss much, unless you're interested in how much of a hormonal monster these drugs are going to turn me into?'

'What, even more so?' he taunted. Bastard.

We both laughed. You had to. It felt as though there was no other option at this point. It was what kept us going, what boosted us on the days when we started to wonder what this was all for and if it would end the way we dreamed. I am so grateful that my husband's sense of humour and ability to mock me even at my lowest ebb always reminded me there was a reason to smile again. To keep on going.

January seemed like the perfect time to at least attempt to be the healthiest version of myself. I mean, the rest of the world was doing it, so why not me too? There were no invites, no catch-ups or events, everyone was burnt out from the festive season. We were starting a building project the following month to extend at the back of our house so I began to use the days to start the sorting process of cupboards and drawers in those rooms that were set to be packed up and walls knocked down. It was strangely cathartic. It felt quite cleansing to be methodically sorting through each space and deciding what to pack and what not to keep. It definitely took my mind off what was beginning to happen in my body.

Chemical changes in our system are a funny old thing; they can take a while to kick in. For me, it was around the seven- to ten-day mark of injections that I really began to feel the brunt of this drug. I felt heavy, tired, like my head was in a fog. No amount of drawer-sorting was about to bring me clarity in this fuzzy mind. I often walked upstairs to get something, only to find myself standing in a room or on the landing wondering what the hell I was there for. It was a fog not dissimilar to the one I had known after Teddy died. Not being able to remember the simplest things and a general feeling of 'stuckness', as I came to call it. I had the occasional headache too. Not often, but when they came they would be an absolute belter. The kind of headache that makes you feel like your head is in a vice, throbbing from the back of your neck right up to your temples. When those took hold, I couldn't look at my laptop or phone screen to get any work done, I had to just relinquish any kind of control I had over the situation and give in to it. Rest was best. I tried to keep my days quiet, enjoy (cold) walks and early nights. It was a simple formula but all I could do to keep myself going, to tick off the days and get to the next stage of this process.

This time we didn't tell anyone what was going on except for my parents. Any friends who asked I told we hadn't started again yet. I wasn't ready for the pressure again. Having to tell everyone in December that we had failed to get off the ground in our first attempt had just felt like another defeat. My heart, and tummy, were bruised. I needed a little time to adjust to these changes, this cycle, before I felt like I could let anyone else back into this process with us. Instead I lay low and used yoga to try to calm my thoughts that were often spinning out of control.

My baseline scan was good! I was switched off and boy did it feel like it. By this point, I felt near numb. It was as if all of the hormones were just gone. The aim of the check-up was to make sure of this and to prep me for the next stage, which meant continuing the daily buserelin injections but adding the stimulation drug back into the mix to fire those ovaries back up again. Things were about to get wild. I was set to do this for the next week and then come back again to begin progress scans on the growing follicles, a part of the protocol I was already familiar with from last time. Everything was good at this point, no worries. I felt ready to get started on the next bit. If anything, I was looking forward to having some kind of hormonal action happening in my body again. I had actually begun to feel listless from the lack of ups and downs that I was used to those monthly cycles giving me.

The next week flew by and I went to see my acupuncturist to help give things a boost, too. I was so fearful of a repeat performance of our last round, I wanted to give my body a fighting chance this time. I was getting quite used to the injections too. More than three weeks in of daily injections and my belly resembled a slightly bruised pear . . . One you might find at the bottom of the fruit bowl that had once been ripe and smooth, but now looked bumpy and brown in places and a little less inviting than it did when you first placed it there amongst its fruity friends. It was becoming hard to try and find a new spot to inject, somewhere fresh that wasn't already recovering from previous injections. I would find myself scouring my belly as part of the nightly ritual, looking for the perfect piece of flesh to pinch and inject. The injections didn't hurt at all now; I didn't even flinch or have to count myself in each time. Weirdly, it was beginning to feel natural. As if I was simply helping my body along in a process it was already able and willing to do. I tried to keep that in my mind – that way my body would go with the flow rather than trying to resist, surely?

The first scan was good. Things *were* happening. I lay there, tense as anything as the internal scanner (dildo wand) worked its magic and I scrawled the numbers and measurements of each follicle she counted on a Post-It note as she read them out. It felt such a relief to know we had got off to another good start. I tried to hold on to this brief moment of positivity, knowing it would be what carried me through the rest of the week between appointments. The nurse seemed happy too, she said that, to be on the safe side, they had kept my stimulation medication fairly low to start with but they were now happy to increase it again for the next few days to give those already-growing follicles a boost. I was happy with this as my side effects at this point had been minimal, the headaches had gone and the only thing I really felt was tired. The remedy for this (as always) was rest and drink plenty of water, so that was what I planned to do.

I saw a couple of close friends for coffee (well, decaf/ herbal tea for me) and let them in on what we were doing. Both were hugely supportive and understanding and they promised not to pry or ask too many questions. I think they could sense how worried I was about the whole thing going completely tits up again after last time. It felt good to tell a couple of people, it was a weight off my chest. I could finally discuss the things that had been weighing so heavily on my mind. I knew they were the right people to tell, too. They wouldn't fuss over me or constantly need updates that I couldn't give.

Never before in my life had I wished more that we had all been designed like Teletubbies (dated reference there, although I am sure those guys have made a comeback?) and we all had screens in our tummies. I just wanted to switch on that screen, take a good old look at what was happening and then I could relax. But alas, my Teletubby alter ego was relaxing elsewhere in a parallel universe while I sat here stressing about my hidden-away ovaries.

The next scan was also good! Result. This time I actually felt elated, as this had been the turning point to not-so-good for us last time. The nurse did say that they were slower than they would have liked so that it would be likely that egg retrieval would be pushed back a few days but I was fine with that. Over the moon, as it happened. The plan was to give those follicles one last boost with a slightly higher dose and reassess. This really was a fine balance – too much and they risked the follicle becoming too big, with an egg too mature for use; too small and we would have a repeat of the last cycle with not enough mature eggs to proceed. I was beginning to understand just what a complex artform it all was. On my last cycle, my one good follicle had indeed been boosted that little too hard, which meant that, even with my trigger shot, it had been too far gone. Instead of releasing an egg (as hoped for), it had gone on to form into a follicular cyst (who knew?). A little surprise that had been waiting for me at my first scan in January that had luckily shrunk down to nothing again during the buserelin phase. There were so many potential complexities, so many bridges you might have to cross. No one, not anyone, was *just doing IVF*. It was a minefield.

After a weekend of resting, guzzling water, continuing with my daily ritual of protein-rich foods and a concoction of fertility-boosting supplements, the day was finally here. Would it be good news this time? Thankfully, it was. Miracles *did* happen. I had 23 follicles of measurable size and egg retrieval was booked for two days' time. I was given my pre-procedure form to fill in and sent on my way with what I hoped was my very last injection, my trigger shot.

Wednesday, 6th February 2019. The biggest day in my calendar in a while. It felt like we had been on such a ride just to make it to this point, but we were finally here. We walked into the hospital at 7:30am that morning waiting for what lay ahead. The main reception area was thronging with people – another 15 couples at least. Obviously a big day in the egg-retrieval world! I panned around the room to rows of nervous faces, everyone bearing the same blank expression of 'What the fuck are we doing here so early?' mixed with a bit of 'How has it come to this?'. Anyone who caught eyes just gestured with a quiet, knowing smile. It was like some weird club. All of us knew exactly what was going on, we were all clinging to that life-raft of IVF that had been flung out in front of us. But who would be lucky today? I often think back and see those faces in my mind, and wonder how many couples who were there that day had a procedure that ended in a successful pregnancy and the birth of a longed-for baby. I have resigned myself to the fact I'll never know but I cling to the hope that it was many of them.

We checked in at the desk and waited for our turn to be collected by a nurse. In time, we were taken up the stairs to the day surgery unit.

'We are very busy with collections today,' the nurse said. I had guessed that by the number of nervous-looking people downstairs. 'It might be a wait, but we'll hope to get you in by lunchtime.'

Blimey. Lunchtime? I hadn't expected it would be that long and I had been nil-by-mouth since last night. As someone who doesn't do well on an empty stomach and whose blood sugar has an awful tendency to come crashing down (a regular fainter in my teenage years!), I tried not to think about it and decided instead to focus on the stack of magazines I had come armed with. I changed into my hospital gown with dressing gown and rather fetching surgical stockings, settled myself onto the bed and prepared to dive into a copy of *Country Homes & Interiors* as my husband watched *Good Morning Britain* on the hospital TV and we chatted about the goings-on that morning. It didn't feel like a hospital, it was comfy and not clinical, quiet and calm. I felt like I was checking in for a mini-break (albeit one that involved no food and the wearing of surgical stockings) and I felt calm. I was trying not to think too much about the sedation itself, as that was the only part that worried me. It had been almost two years since my last general anaesthetic, when my consultant had had to retrieve the remnants of something left in my uterus after the loss of our last baby. I tried not to let my thoughts wander back there, to how scared I had been. I wanted this to be a new experience, a positive one. The cosy room and magazines were definitely helping.

I also forgot that my husband had an important part to play today. Those eggs, if collected, weren't going to miraculously fertilise themselves. He had to provide a sample which would be delivered to the embryology lab and used later that day in the same Petri dish (I imagine?) as the eggs. It was the first time in this entire process that I felt sorry for him; it all felt so personal and a bit embarrassing. I mean, at least I got to be knocked out for my bit, I didn't have to feel an ounce of embarrassment! The nurse who talked him through the process was really understanding and made a lot of jokes about the process in among her instructions of where and what time to deliver his little bag that contained the sample pot. She was also very kind in saying that because they were so busy that day he didn't have to make his way to the special room they provided for this process and that the hospital room ensuite would suffice. I resisted the temptation to hammer on the door and shout 'How you getting on in there?' Luckily it was another of those times where we found inappropriate jokes and laughter the best way through!

After several hours of waiting and one M&S dash for my husband (who was apparently starving, poor thing), we were ready for my turn. I had given strict instructions prior to said M&S run regarding all the snack foods I needed to be ready upon my return and when I felt well enough to eat again after the sedation. I was dreaming of iced buns and an ice-cold juice, perhaps a sandwich? Suddenly all I could think about were snack foods! And then I was finally being wheeled into the room for sedation.

There were about four people in there – a nurse, a couple of anaesthetists and a consultant. The usual procedures of checking they had the right person began: asking my name and date of birth and double-checking the band around my wrist. Much like the clinic waiting room of people being ushered from room to room for their appointments, this was an efficient operation – everyone had their place and each cog knew exactly what it was doing. I lay there trying to guess what number I was on the list today and how many eggs had already been successfully extracted out into the world. The next thing I knew, the needle was in my arm, I was being asked if I had any holidays planned for that year and the familiar rush was tingling through my veins and over my head. Gone.

'How many did you get?'

These are the first words I remember slurring to the nurse in the recovery room as I came around. My mind had obviously not switched off even though I had been out cold. Keen to know the outcome I pressed her straight away!

'I'm not allowed to tell you that. You'll get a visit from the embryologist when you're out of recovery and back in your room. My job is to make sure you're OK and get you back there,' she said with a smile.

She must have been used to keen-beans like me. Waking up desperate to know what it had all been for. Five, ten, fifteen maybe? I just knew I couldn't wait much longer to find out. As they wheeled me back into the room, I was greeted by my husband's gentle smiling face once more. A welcome sight, as I was feeling rather groggy.

'How are you feeling, my love?'

'Like I've just been hit by a bus . . . but hungry,' I replied.

Just as I was cracking into my first Lucozade Sport (gotta get those electrolytes up!) a tall, elegant and happy-looking lady came into the room after a couple of knocks on the door.

'Mr and Mrs Wright, I'm from the embryology team and I'm here to tell you about how today's procedure has gone.'

Both of us held our breath and the room fell silent. Hanging on her every word, we waited as she began to speak again.

'We've collected ten mature eggs today. That's a really nice number. So, well done. Make sure you get plenty of rest and we'll give you a call tomorrow to let you know how many have successfully fertilised.'

We were egg-static! (Sorry. Bad, but too easy.) It was a mix of relief and joy. Everything now lay in the lap of the universe and we would hold our breath again until tomorrow and hope that we got a good outcome. Just as soon as you have flown down one drop of the rollercoaster you find yourself on the steep ascent back to the top, teetering on the precipice of the next drop, waiting for your stomach to experience that familiar lurch as you freefall to the next step of the process.

A couple of hours (and a lot of snacks) later we were ready to go home. I was beginning to feel a little sore as the sedation and painkillers wore off. We left armed with more painkillers, a number to call in case of emergency and a new bag of drugs – this time, progesterone pessaries. The pessaries were to start later that day, to mimic the rise of progesterone in the body after ovulation and hopefully help support the implantation of any embryo that made its way back in there. They could be inserted 'back or front' but I was instructed that back would be preferable in this instance, given that I had just had a procedure through the front entrance and it would reduce any risk of infection if I used the back. (To anyone who has completely lost the thread here I am referring to inserting pessaries up my arse as opposed to up my vagina but I was just trying to keep things low-key out of fear that my dad or my brothers may one day read these words and never be able to look me in the eye again. Oh well, damage is done.)

I hobbled back to the car and felt every bump of the journey home. When we got back, I hurried upstairs for a warm shower and to put my softest pyjamas on. I hunkered down in bed as it was dark by 5pm and so easy to feel like the day had already come to an end. I wanted it to be over. I was, after all, hanging on for tomorrow's phone call.

As I sat at my dressing table not long after 8am the next morning, my silent phone began flashing next to me. *Unknown caller ID*. My mouth was dry and I could barely speak as I answered. My heart thumped as I listened to the friendly voice on the end of the line. It was the same lady who had greeted us so cheerfully yesterday.

'Good news,' she said. 'Three of your eggs have fertilised so we have three embryos looking good. The nurses will call you later to arrange your transfer. Most likely for Monday but perhaps before if things aren't looking as positive.'

Positive? Well, this didn't feel very fucking positive. Yesterday we had ten healthy eggs, today we have just three embryos? I didn't like these statistics. As I put the phone down and before I began to completely lose myself in my own thoughts, I realised I should probably call my husband who was already at work.

'Just three,' I said flatly, defeated once more.

'Elle, it only takes one. Remember that.'

He was right, so right, and I *knew* that. I had just become so used to things looking great and then slowly but surely the good news parts ebbing away and suddenly being left with nothing. This was how this process was looking so far: Monday saw 23 follicles, yesterday ten eggs, today just three embryos. So what awaited us tomorrow? Zero? I couldn't bear to even contemplate it. Instead I busied myself with more packing in the house and took Boris, our pug, for a long walk in the cold February air. The very first signs of spring were popping up and the birds were singing. I tried to focus on the positives. We still had three and new life was trying to burst through the cold snap of winter all around me.

When the call came the next morning, I could barely bring myself to answer it. Time stood still as I listened. We still had all three. I couldn't believe it.

'You'll be going ahead with a transfer of one on Monday. Only if anything deteriorates or changes over the weekend will you hear from us.'

You could tell she had delivered those words a thousand times before, that she was just doing her job. I couldn't help but thank her endlessly though, she had made my day – my week, my year! We were one step closer and just had to make it through another weekend with no bad news. I was crossing everything, there was nothing else left to cross. *No phone calls over the weekend*. I wished with every cell of my being that my phone would not ring. Most of the time I couldn't pick it up to look just in case. It was a torturous waiting game, another climb on the rollercoaster.

The pessaries had been going well with no side effects and I was feeling glad to be free from injections. I had spent the days since egg retrieval eating nourishing foods that I thought would help to thicken my lining and warm my uterus, making it a comfortable haven for any budding baby in the making.

Monday was transfer day and we were all set. I have to say, of all the appointments that we attended, this was perhaps the most underwhelming. I don't know what I had expected, to be honest – a big fanfare celebration, a confetti cannon, perhaps? It felt like a bit of an anti-climax being led into a soulless little box of a room with a bed in the centre and something that resembled a 1970s dining-room hatch on one wall. As the nurse got me settled onto the bed, trousers removed and modesty intact under a disposable sheet, the consultant began to talk through the procedure as the cheery and familiar face of the embryologist appeared from behind the doors of the hatch.

It was all rather surreal. We could see as the embryo was transferred into the dish, ready for its final destination. It was being shown to us on a screen in the room and we watched as it hopped and jiggled around on the screen looking like a full moon in a Petri dish. Last checks were made, confirming our names, dates of birth and other details were correct before this little one was transferred. I was lying flat now, knees bent, shaking. In many ways, it was much like so many of the procedures I had faced so far – but this one was *different*. The consultant picked up the embryo in an instrument that looked much like a medical turkey baster to me and the little moon disappeared from the screen. The next thing I knew I felt a slightly scratchy, cramping sensation for just a few seconds and then . . .

'There we go. All done.'

See, I told you. An anti-climax or what? Not so much as a flake of confetti came down from the sky. It had been wonderful, though, seeing that little moon on the screen, that little chance, our chance, now floating around inside me.

As I dressed myself and sat on the side of the bed listening to the nurse go over our aftercare and instructions of when to test, I felt a strange rush come over me. It sounds cheesy but it was as if everything had changed in that moment. I had walked in just one person but was leaving with something special on board.

Her words echoed in my ears as she repeated how I should look after myself for the next two weeks.

'Because don't forget, you're now technically pregnant, until proven otherwise.'

I held on to that magical prospect as we walked out of the doors into the new spring air.

Chapter 9

Good News or Bad?

MY HANDS WERE SHAKING AS I SAT IN THE BATHROOM WAITING FOR THE RESULT; FEELING AS THOUGH I WAS ON A PRECIPICE. Preparing to fall one way or the other. Would it be good news, or more bad? I had spent the last two weeks looking for signs and symptoms, taunting myself with *Oh, that must mean I am* and *Oh well, that definitely means it hasn't worked then.* I swerved from elation to despair on a daily basis. Trying not to worry or think about something when that particular something is (or is not) going on inside your own body is an impossible task.

These two weeks had been filled with all manner of distractions. Shopping trips, work commitments, coffee dates, anything that made me feel happy – all of the things I had cleared from my diary for the previous seven weeks. I binged on TV programmes that made me laugh (I never, ever binge watch anything), I took daily walks, enjoyed gentle yoga, read every single helpful online blog related to the two-week wait, while simultaneously trying not to lose my mind.

My meals were warming; I avoided cold drinks and ice like it might kill me the very moment it touched my lips. I tried everything I could within my own realms of 'doable' to make this happen for us. Shouldering the guilt of this not working wasn't worth contemplating; I already felt like this was all on me. Silly, I know, it takes two to tango as they say, but when *you* are the one who has been trusted to carry that little embryo and make a safe, warm and welcoming home for it, it feels that way. I was hoping all of my efforts hadn't been in vain. I had read success stories aplenty, and heart-breaking ones too. When you are in the middle of that waiting game it's hard not to fixate on which camp you might fall into. You want to believe it will happen for you, this time, but at the same time you daren't get carried away on a dream that has yet come to fruition. After all, we all know that the fall always feels so much harder when you have so much further to tumble.

I had been to see Emma Cannon in these two weeks too. I booked a treatment with her for the day after my transfer. I didn't know anyone else who would be able to lift my spirits and encourage positive belief quite like she could. I had read that having acupuncture in the 24–48 hours after transfer could really help to improve the chances of the embryo implanting, so for me it felt like a no-brainer. We had come this far, why wouldn't I try one last thing to make this happen? One final throw of the dice.

I found it difficult to relax in that treatment session, impossible even. Knowing that little embryo was floating around in there, looking for somewhere to settle. Had its fate already been decided? But Emma was, as expected, just the tonic I needed that day. It wasn't just about having the treatment with her, it was the wisdom she imparted and the words she used. It was refreshing to speak with someone who truly believed in the power of the human body; in the power of *my* body. Something that had become increasingly difficult for me to believe in of late. Her words were calming and reassuring. The needles tingled as she twiddled them in my tummy and I felt a rush of energy swell in my belly.

As I was leaving, Emma said, 'Who do you think might be in there? Do you like to think of it as Teddy's soul returning or someone new?'

It was a question, like so many of hers, that I hadn't been expecting. Yet without so much of a flinch of hesitation I responded, 'Someone completely new. A really special soul.'

'That's exactly what I felt too,' she said with a knowing smile.

I left with a sense of calm and happiness. All of the worry and anxiety of the weeks before seemed to wash away. It was the best way I could have started that two-week wait.

However, no matter how much I tried to keep them topped up, those feelings of positivity and calm that I left Emma's office with slowly chipped away over the next two weeks, no matter how much I tried to top it up.

Now I was sitting in the bathroom again, waiting for the culmination of the last two months. Every injection, every appointment, every dalliance with the dildo wand, every single tear and worried thought – it all came down to this. I tested a day early (I know, rebel). I couldn't wait and I didn't see the difference a day would make at this late stage. I had read a lot online about testing the trigger shot out of your system (it contains HCG pregnancy hormone, so could give a false positive). Many women seemed to test every day from transfer until they knew the trigger was gone, then continue to test until tests turn positive again. I didn't think I could handle that process – I found the torment of peeing on sticks bad enough so I wanted to do it as little as humanly possible.

I'd had a day-five embryo transferred and it would have taken a few days for it to implant successfully (if that was going to be the case) and then a further 48 hours for my body to begin producing pregnancy hormone that would be detectable in a blood test and urine test. This point felt like a 'safe' day to test. It may not have been *the* day marked on my treatment plan, but I felt ready. . .

Two lines. I was seeing things, surely? We had been here before after the first round of Clomid, so I couldn't bring myself to believe it. It felt like a miracle. These lines weren't faint though, they weren't barely there, they didn't need holding to a window or asking for a second opinion. They were two, dark, ruby-red lines staring straight back at me. I was shaking like never before. I couldn't call the clinic and tell them or they would know I had cheated and caved a day early. Instead I sent a photo to my husband. He responded immediately.

'See, I told you. It only takes one. Xxxxx'

A rush of excitement, relief, love and pride swelled through me. I could feel it in every cell. Suddenly, in that moment, it all felt worth it. We *were* those lucky ones, the ones whose first embryo transfer ended in a baby. My mind swung back to that waiting room on egg retrieval day, to the scared faces of all of those other couples, and I couldn't help but wonder if there was anyone else who was getting to feel this way too.

I spent the rest of the day feeling as if I was floating around in a blissful bubble of elation and disbelief. I wanted to shout it from the roof tops but at the same time was too scared to tell a soul. I couldn't wait for Nico to get home from work so that I could give him the biggest hug. I just wanted to be with him, to share in this moment of happiness. It felt so strange that we had to spend the day apart but it was just a Thursday, like any other Thursday. The day moved at a snail's pace as I waited for the moment I heard him turn his key in the door.

'I'll do another test tomorrow though,' I said, as if to reassure myself. 'Just to be sure.'

And I did. In fact, I bought myself a fancy digital pack, just to be doubly sure. Not even yesterday's result was enough to stop me panicking as I waited for the result of the second test. Much to my surprise, it was better than I thought. It read '2–3 weeks pregnant'. This was good news; it must have meant that my HCG levels were already high. I had only expected to see a result of 1–2 weeks, so this felt like the extra reassurance I had craved. It was now Friday, so our official test day. My parents were on their way to Cornwall for my mum's birthday break and, seeing as they were two of the few people who knew about the result we were waiting for, I had promised to text my mum and tell her either way. Although, we had pre-empted the possible emotions with either result and decided that a simple thumbs up or thumbs down emoji would be the best way for me to communicate the news. I tapped out a thumbs up and pressed send. Although she always pretended to play it cool in these situations, I guessed she must have been waiting phone-in-hand, as within a matter of seconds a reply came back. A string of thumbs ups, hearts, crying faces and a long string of kisses. Followed by another message saying, simply, 'Love you. Xxxx'.

I would speak to her later but for now I needed to stare endlessly at that glaringly positive result and call the clinic to tell them our good news. They were just as I had expected they would be. I got to speak to the nurse I had seen in my many appointments, who congratulated me in a warm and genuine way. I almost forgot how wonderful it must be for them to receive good news after all of their efforts; they must really feel it too. She booked me for a six-week viability scan at the clinic, which was two weeks away.

Another two-week wait. I couldn't cope. Suddenly I was thrown back into the waiting game and worry began to take over. I understood why it was pointless seeing us before that point: no scan would be able to see anything at all. The point of the viability scan would be to determine that there was a developing pregnancy in the correct place and, after that, we would be passed back over into the care of the main hospital trust for the remainder of our pregnancy. It made complete sense. The nurse instructed me to carry on with the progesterone pessaries until my next visit (what a continuous joy those had been!), and reminded me to rest, drink plenty of water and enjoy this happy moment.

Oh, I did. That day, I was on cloud nine. Suddenly, all of the worries of the past two and a half years felt like they had led us to this moment. I remember taking a cheesy selfie in the mirror, proudly holding up my test result of 2–3 weeks. Beaming at myself. It felt like an impossible dream had been achieved.

It was the next morning that I felt the bubble begin to burst. Not a full-blown *pop* as such, more of a gradual leak (and so far more worrying). The day started as any other weekend would, sitting up in bed and chatting to my husband, enjoying my cup of tea and, this time, a new-found happiness. We had plans to go to friends' that day to watch the rugby and have lunch together. I went to the bathroom later that morning.

'I'm bleeding.'

'What do you mean? How much?' came Nico's reply from outside the door.

'Not a lot. Not like proper blood or anything, but it's there.'

I felt sick. I'm pretty sure the colour and any positive glow drained from me in that moment. It was replaced with a feeling of being completely and utterly petrified at what was happening. I didn't know what to do. It was Saturday, the clinic was closed. I felt like I was being melodramatic calling their emergency line. I mean, *was* this an emergency? It wasn't even like I was properly bleeding, just spotting, but it was enough to plant a seed of doubt firmly in my mind. We decided to go about the day as planned but every bathroom trip came with a new wave of worry and me checking and double-checking to see if there was more blood. Sometimes it was there, sometimes it wasn't. I tried to put it to the back of my mind; we would deal with it on Monday.

I have no idea now, looking back, why I thought waiting until Monday would make it better, might make it go away, somehow. The worry was constant and deep-set, like a dark cloud hanging heavily over the remainder of the weekend. What had started as the happiest we had both felt in a long while had quickly spun into a weekend of panic. I lost myself in Google searches. 'Four weeks pregnant and spotting blood.' Reams of answers, stories and forums came up. I skimmed a few, only fuelling my panic further.

Monday came around and the blood was still there – not always, not every time, but it was there. I waited until early afternoon, until I couldn't shoulder the worry any longer, and called the hospital Early Pregnancy Unit.

They were brilliant. Luckily, I got through to a nurse who remembered me from previous visits.

'Come straight in,' she said. 'I can't promise we'll be able to see anything on a scan as it's so early but we can certainly get one of the doctors to have a look at you and we can run some blood tests to check your HCG.'

I went immediately. The afternoon passed in a blur of waiting and explaining everything and more waiting and then, finally, a scan with a doctor. She was lovely, so empathetic, and she tried her best to reassure me.

'I can't see anything yet but it is so early going by your IVF dates. Are you in any pain?'

'Not noticeably,' I replied. 'Just the usual twinges and cramps I would have thought were normal right now?' I didn't know. Was I in pain? Mentally and emotionally, yes. Could I feel physical pain in there though? It sounds silly but I didn't know. I was numb from it all.

'Well, we've run some blood tests. I'll have the results of those in the morning so that should give us a clearer picture. In the meantime, you go home and rest and please call us if that bleeding becomes any heavier or if you are experiencing any pain.'

She was right, there was little they could do right now. With nothing on the screen and no blood test to go on, no one would have any clue what was going on in there. It was another waiting game and I was very used to those by now.

It turned out to be the shortest waiting game I had ever experienced, as my phone rang at 7:30am the following morning. It was the doctor from the hospital and I was silent as I listened to her words. What came next is a blur. She explained that my blood HCG was really high for that point in a pregnancy and for them not to be seeing anything. She told me she suspected an ectopic pregnancy.

The words rang around my head. *Surely not?* She asked me if I could head back to the hospital, this morning, immediately. I called Nico and asked him to leave work and meet me there. I called my mum in tears and apologised to her for letting everyone down, *again.* I remembered in that moment that it was my mum's birthday and realised I had ruined that too.

As instructed, I made my way back to the hospital and was taken straight to a room in the EPU. Two consultants and a nurse were waiting to look after me. I filled in forms, blinded by tears pricking in my eyes as they took blood and put a cannula in my hand. I was then taken back to the same room from yesterday to be re-scanned. They could see something there, between my right ovary and my tube. My prickling eyes turned to sobs just as Nico arrived. The consultants were kind and kept trying their best to reassure us, even once it was clear that it wasn't good news. One of them told us about his and his wife's struggle to have a baby, about their IVF treatment and their losses. 'It never leaves you,' he said and I could see that he was holding back tears as he looked after us.

We were taken to a ward and I was put on a drip as I hadn't eaten since the previous night and couldn't have anything to eat or drink. The ward and cubicle were identical to the one I was in when Teddy stopped breathing. I began to panic that I was going to die here too.

Lunchtime came and went and the afternoon passed by. The consultant came every couple of hours to apologise for the wait and I begged them to let this be over. I was taken down to theatre at 7pm. More people crowded over me as I waited for the anaesthetic (I remembered that I *still* hate anaesthetic). I was shaking as the nurse squeezed my hand to try to comfort me. I felt that familiar rush up my arm and my neck.

I woke up late that evening and saw the consultant. It had gone 9pm; she had stayed to make sure she could do the operation herself. *What a wonderful human*, I thought to myself.

She said, 'We have some good news.' There was no ectopic pregnancy after all.

'We've left everything in there and I will speak to you in the morning about what we do next.'

I felt relieved, overjoyed and, then, confused beyond measure. They wheeled me back to the ward where my husband was waiting for me. Tears streamed down my face but I don't even know why anymore! Nico had to leave as it was late. I didn't sleep, I just snacked instead, in case not being starving might bring more clarity to this situation. I doubted it. The hazy feeling from the anaesthetic made me want to vomit, though.

The next morning it all felt like a bad dream, but it wasn't. I was still there, in a hospital bed. I hadn't slept, just lay awake all night wondering how all of this had happened in a matter of hours. I lifted the sheets and my gown and, staring back at me, was a set of dressings over what I imagined to be a set of jazzy new abdominal scars. War wounds; more proof of this emotional and physical journey.

Nico arrived back not long after 8am and the consultant joined us soon after. I sipped on an Earl Grey tea my husband had bought for me as I listened to the doctors. They didn't have a plan, as such. We were to wait a week. They wanted to re-scan and see if there was anything to be seen then. They would discharge me today and I was to watch for any more bleeding. Although there could be a little more bleeding from the operation I had just had. I was confused; how was I to know which was which?

I left after a couple more hours, battered and bruised. I was worried that the anaesthetic and morphine from yesterday would have done more harm if indeed there was a baby still in there, trying to survive. Had I just made this a million times worse because I worried too early? Should I have gone to the EPU on Monday at all? The guilt started to set in again.

It wasn't ectopic, we knew that now, but was this good news, or bad?

Chapter 10

When Lightning Strikes Twice

AS I GOT HOME THAT AFTERNOON, THE TEARS STARTED TO FLOW UNCONTROLLABLY. The doctor had told me to carry on with the progesterone pessaries, just in case, but this felt like a pointless task, as if I was hanging on to the last shred of hope, willing for this to all be OK. I was sore, literally and figuratively. My phone was buzzing constantly with concerned messages from friends and family asking if I was OK. I didn't have the energy to answer, I couldn't bring myself to explain that we were in the middle of another unknown. I sent a text to a couple of best friends but that was the best I could manage. I knew I couldn't face phone calls or FaceTimes with anyone. I didn't know what to tell them because we didn't know ourselves. This was a waiting game, the worst kind of waiting game. I had to try not to worry for a whole week. The impossible task.

Suffice to say, I fell down a Google rabbit hole with almost immediate effect after returning home. Reading up on bleeding in early pregnancy, miscarriage, missed miscarriage and more, I felt as though I was armed with my baby-loss bingo card, adding a nice big splodge upon each square with every pregnancy experience so far. Was this some kind of sick joke? Surely this couldn't happen after everything else? I frantically Googled (other search engines available) statistics on repeat loss, miscarriage after IVF, miscarriage by age of mother – anything I could think of that might bring me some clarity, some answers in this limbo-land of waiting. Nothing did, of course. It was as if that week moved in painful slow-motion, scan day edging towards us while I watched the seconds ticking down on the clock.

I had to go to the hospital on my own that morning. Nico had to be at work again and my mum had offered to drive to and come with me but I had told her there wasn't any need. I was trying to be stoic and strong. I have no idea why. I think perhaps because I didn't want to place any of this anguish of waiting and the inevitable disappointment on anyone else. At best, I was still only five and a half weeks pregnant, even though this treatment cycle and the time afterwards had been months already. It was now March. The perfect time for new beginnings.

I was taken straight into the scan room in the EPU, no waiting this time. It was a different consultant who saw me, silent as she scanned, and the nurse from last week squeezed my hand. I watched on, staring into the blank abyss of the black screen, looking for clues, for signs of life. All I could see was a blob, a little blob.

'I'm sorry,' the consultant said softly as she put her hand on my leg and tilted her head as she spoke. 'It looks as though there was a developing pregnancy there, I can see the sac, but it's not developing any longer. It's what we call a missed miscarriage. We can help you manage this.'

These were words I had expected after a week of searching for answers on my own, they were words that already felt familiar in their tone and delivery. But I still felt shock. That wave of sadness rising towards me, waiting to pull me under again.

'How can you be sure?' I asked, wanting certainty.

'By this time, we might expect to see more but there is nothing.'

Nothing. Of course, there was nothing. All these months of preparing, the weeks of injections, the tears, the hope and secrecy that turned into celebration, all manifested into *nothing*.

Tears began running down my face as if someone had turned a tap on. I lay there motionless on the bed, expecting someone to say something else. No one spoke for a moment as the consultant cleaned the scanner and began to tap some notes into her screen. The nurse ushered me to get dressed again. I returned to the bed and sat on the side, listening as the consultant spoke again.

'As I said, there are ways we can manage it. You can take medication today to help end the pregnancy and encourage miscarriage naturally or we can arrange a D&C procedure and I can get you on a list for tomorrow. With your history of retained products of pregnancy, I might recommend the latter, although we will explain the risks of both to you.'

I couldn't take in what was happening. Her words washed over me in a blur. I was hearing them but I didn't know what to say. Before I knew it, another senior nurse appeared; she was asking me to go and sit in another room. She explained that they would take blood to look at my HCG (pregnancy hormone) levels again and compare them to last week's when I had been discharged after surgery.

'I'll get the relevant paperwork for you to sign and then we can get you onto that operating list for tomorrow . . .'

'No,' I replied. 'I don't want to.'

The words seemed to leave my mouth before I could stop them. I didn't know what I was saying, all I knew was that I wasn't about to accept that this was over. If my week of Google research had taught me anything, it was that miracles could, and did, happen. Perhaps not for me but for some people they had. I wanted a second opinion. I asked the nurse what the IVF doctor at the other hospital had said about it. After all, he worked between both and I was certain he would have known what had been going on for the past week. She said she didn't know if there had been any communication.

It was at that point I decided I would leave that day without signing anything. I let her take my bloods and agreed that she could call me tomorrow to discuss my options further but I told her I wouldn't be making any decisions there and then. I needed time to think and to accept what I had just been told. My body had managed to hold on to the pregnancy so far, whether it was still developing or not, so I was hoping it could hold on another twenty-four hours while I got my mental and emotional shit together enough to make an informed decision.

I remember feeling a rush of relief run through me as I walked out of the hospital. I didn't want to be railroaded into deciding that day, in that little room. As I drove home, I decided to do two things. I called the IVF clinic and asked them if they knew what was going on. They did not. After a brief conversation, I agreed to go in that afternoon for a scan with them. Secondly, I called my mum. I told her what had just happened at the hospital and that I *did* need her. I needed a second opinion, I needed support and I needed a hug.

I went home, waited for my mum and called my husband to let him know what I had done. It didn't feel right sitting in that hospital room, being asked to make that decision about this longed-for baby, without him. He agreed that he thought I had done the right thing in not being hasty. It had been a whirlwind week of waiting and I had already had one unexpected surgery. I wasn't about to commit to another without at least having the time to think it over.

Later that afternoon, I drove over to the IVF clinic with my mum. I was so glad I had someone with me. It felt completely different to how I had felt that morning, going in alone, trying desperately to prop up all of these emotions by myself. She was the calming voice I needed. Whatever happened, she would be there to take me home afterwards and we would work through it. In all of the months I had been going to the IVF clinic, it was the first time she had accompanied me and I only wish it had been in better circumstances. She, like me, also marvelled at the thousand smiling babies on the walls that greeted us. I knew how much she wanted another grandchild and how much she wanted this for us and I only wished I could give that to her.

I walked into a room that now felt comfortable and familiar – it was where I had been coming for all of my follicle tracking scans during treatment. The same friendly nurse sonographer was there to look after me. Even if this was still bad news, I felt as though I could handle it with her there and my mum by my side. Before she started, she asked me to explain what had happened over the last ten days – everything from when I had called them about my positive test to why I was sitting there now.

I explained in detail as she and the other nurse listened, open-mouthed at the story that unfolded.

They couldn't understand why there hadn't been communication between the two hospitals and she said she felt that a secondary scan was a good place to start before we moved forward with anything. She began scanning, both her and the other nurse staring at the screen intently, just as I had been doing this morning. I chose not to look this time. I was trying to read the expression on their faces instead. My eyes darted between their faces and my mum's, as everyone looked for a flicker of life.

'Well, I wouldn't say we could definitively call it a missed miscarriage at this stage. You are so early still. I do a lot of early scans here and sometimes this is all we can see. There's a sac and potentially what looks like the start of a foetal pole, but no heartbeat. I would say we need to give it more time before we do anything.'

I felt a smile beginning to creep across my face. 'Thank you,' I said.

She had re-ignited a glimmer of hope, one that had felt long gone in the morning's appointment. So, what now? I asked. I was starting to feel like I asked that question on repeat at the moment. (Perhaps it could become my slogan with an accompanying range of merch?)

'I'd say we need to wait another week. I also need to communicate this with the other hospital and send these scan images and my report to your consultant there. Once we have re-scanned next week then we'll be able to give you a definitive answer, as that would have been your six-week viability scan anyway.'

Her words were reassuring and I immediately felt as though things would be more straightforward from here. I hadn't bled in a few days, so that had to be a good thing. The advice, again, was to rest and wait and to continue with the progesterone pessaries. I went to the pharmacy to collect more.

'Well, that's better news than this morning?' said my mum as we made our way back to the car. Almost as though she was asking a question as opposed to stating a fact. I suppose because neither of us knew. Was it good? Was it *better* news? Or, was it delaying the inevitable once more?

My mum decided to stay for a few days and look after me while I fell down a few more Google rabbit holes . . . My husband promised that he'd make it to the next scan so that we could make any decision together. The weekend and the rest of the week felt longer than the last. There is no way to distract yourself. No amount of long walks, watching rom-coms or eating your favourite food will wash away the worry in that waiting time. It was like the two-week wait, but on steroids. Still, we tried our best. I didn't think it was possible but time seemed to slow down even further in that week.

I felt strangely positive the morning we walked back into the IVF clinic for the latest update on the 'Pregnant or Not?' mystery. I have no idea why – perhaps that last scan had helped me to see that there *might* still be a chance, however tiny. I just wanted an answer and for this bizarre limbo of waiting to be over. My husband squeezed my hand as we sat and waited. The usual morning television blasted out of the TV as people stared blankly up at it. No one spoke.

When we were finally called in, I could feel my palms starting to sweat and heard a notable shake in my voice as I greeted the same nurse sonographer from last week. She was so thoughtful, asking me how I had managed the last week and saying she hoped it had not just been full of worry. She and I both knew it had been.

She began scanning. I couldn't look at the screen, but I noticed that Nico was. I glanced up and saw the blob again (that's all I could describe it as). She was taking her time, scanning and investigating what felt like every corner of my uterus. Then:

'I'm sorry. I can't see any changes from the last scan. It almost looks like it might be getting smaller but it's not developing as we would have expected. Sometimes the body can do that, it tries to re-absorb it.'

'OK. It's OK,' I remember saying. 'At least we know now. Thank you.'

I didn't really know why I was thanking her, probably for her genuine compassion and the fact that she had just delivered such a devastating blow in such a kind way.

'We'll need to refer you straight back to the consultant at the hospital so that they can make an immediate plan to assist you with the management of this.'

I dusted myself off as I climbed of the bed and slipped back into my (now pretty tight from all of the progesterone) jeans.

'OK,' I replied. 'I'll call them, and the EPU. I'll let them know.'

She agreed to give me copies of her scan images, this week and last, and an accompanying report from both. This should be all I needed to scan and send to the consultant's secretary that day.

Nico and I walked out, hand in hand again, and barely uttered a word on the journey home. There didn't seem like there was anything left to say.

Within two days, I was back at the hospital for 7:30am, checked into the day surgery unit ready for a D&C procedure. A D&C, standing for dilation and curettage, is the surgical management of a miscarriage, generally used when the pregnancy hasn't, or can't, pass itself naturally. The same kind consultant who had operated on me two weeks previously came to see me for my pre-operative checks, along with my usual consultant. They seemed genuinely gutted for us and both put a reassuring hand on mine as they sat beside me on the bed and explained what they would be doing that day. I could barely speak.

I was being wheeled on a bed into the anaesthetic room before 9am I think they wanted this ordeal to be over as quickly as I did so I must have been first on their list that day. It felt so strange being wheeled on a bed down those corridors again. I just hoped it would be easier this time. Oh, the irony that that had been my last thought as I drifted off . . .

When I woke up, I saw the face of my consultant immediately. She was standing over me, almost as if she had been willing me to wake up sooner. *This was different*, I thought. I was used to waking up in recovery, usually surrounded by nurses who I didn't recognise. Why was she here?

'I'm so sorry.'

Oh fuck, those words again.

'I didn't do the procedure. By that, I mean I couldn't go ahead with the procedure . . .'

Hang on a minute, what on earth was she saying? I was barely conscious and her words weren't making any sense at all. I remember her holding a screen up in front of me with an image. What exactly was I looking at?

'As you know, we were doing the procedure under the guidance of ultrasound, as I wanted to ensure that we saw everything and removed everything, so that you didn't have any repeat problems of what happened with your last medical termination. Well, we were about to start and I was scanning with the ultrasound, and then we had to stop.'

She seemed to almost pause herself at this point and I had absolutely no clue what would come next. 'Because what we saw on the screen were two sacs. There are two potential pregnancies, not one.'

I stared at the onscreen image she was showing me again. Well, fucking hell, *two* blobs. I honestly did not know what was real and what was a dream in this moment. I also didn't know whether to laugh or cry. I had gone to sleep in the hope this would all be over when I woke, and now *this*. I had never expected *this*.

The rest of my time in recovery passed in a haze. I was eager to get back to the ward, I needed to speak to my husband, now. I needed to know if he knew. As they eventually wheeled me back onto the ward, I saw him sitting there and the expression on his face. He knew.

As the nurse and porter left it was an eternity before one of us said something.

'Well . . .' I started.

He began chuckling, the kind of laugh that he and I both do when we are completely out of our depth and have no idea what on earth is going on anymore.

'Aren't you going to say anything?' I asked.

'Elle, I don't know what to say. This is the third time in two weeks we've been told we've lost a baby. Your second operation. And now I've just been told it might be twins?!'

His face was as confused as I had imagined mine looked when the consultant had spoken to me.

'I know. You definitely couldn't make this shit up,' I said. 'I'm exhausted.'

We held hands and smiled at one another. I could tell he didn't know whether laughter or tears were called for right now either. He had already gone and fetched me an Earl Grey, though; he knew so well what would fuel my recovery! This was utter madness but, in this moment, a cup of tea was the little bit of normal that I needed.

It wasn't long before the doctors returned, explaining they would take more bloods before they discharged me to see whether my HCG levels were still rising. I didn't even ask my usual 'What now?'. I didn't have the energy so let them continue.

The plan was to re-scan, again, in five days. Five more days of waiting. You would have thought I would have been used to this protocol by now.

When we got home that day, I didn't know what to say to my family when they called, or my friends. How could I explain something that I didn't understand myself? I didn't even know this was a *thing*. If my head had been spinning before, it was almost in orbit right now. For the first time in weeks, I even turned my back on doctor Google; we had well and truly fallen out. No forum or online medical paper could help me now. We were in uncharted territory, even for the doctors who were treating me. Even they seemed confused! I had no choice but to wait.

During those five days, my HCG must have sky-rocketed. I have never felt so sick and nauseous. I could barely lift my head from the pillow as the room span. It felt like all of the worst hangovers of my twenties rolled into one. Beige food was my only friend. The thirst was intense too – I was putting three glasses of water on my bedside table each night. Something didn't feel right. My mind wandered in and out of thoughts – from no babies at all, to the possibility of *two*. Were rainbow babies really like buses? You wait, and you wait, and you wait, and then . . .

Surely, we couldn't be *that* lucky, after all of this? We knew we only had the one embryo transferred, one flickering moon on the monitor that day. So how, *why*, had this happened? I knew Google would probably have the answers, or at least some ideas, but we definitely still weren't speaking. Instead I spent the days not leaving the house, terrified about losing now not one, but *two* more babies.

We were back in the scanning room in the EPU at the main hospital again.

Time felt like it stood still as I lay there on the bed, hoping this would be the last of the waiting games over. I don't think I will ever forget that final scan. Those two empty sacs on the screen next to one another. The way the consultant apologised and looked as though she was going to cry too. The way she placed her hand on my leg as she delivered the news we had all been dreading. The way my husband squeezed my hand so tightly and the hug that the nurse gave me before she took us through to another room to discuss what would happen next.

I never would have expected twins, I never would have dared dream of them, but seeing them there on the screen made it all the more real, what we had just lost. The consultant said, 'I wish I had been able to give you both some happy news. I really do.' So did I, more than she will ever know. All of the waiting over those weeks, all of the hope, everything seemed to come crashing down, for the final time, in that moment.

'I'm sorry,' I said to my husband as we got back into the car.

'Elle, please, this is no one's fault. Least of all yours.'

Even though his words were heartfelt and powerful, I couldn't help but feel sorry. Sorry for him, for myself, for that little embryo who had turned into the possibility of two little beings. For all of the doctors and nurses over those weeks who had held our hands and held on to that hope for us when we felt like we couldn't anymore. I felt sorry for all of it, and I felt completely empty.

I was back in hospital two days later. The third check-in for surgery. Hopefully, the final time for a while. It's really coming to something when the anaesthetist actually recognises you as a regular customer.

'Back so soon?' he joked as I was wheeled yet again into surgery. It was the only thing that made me truly laugh that day. He was lovely but I really hoped I didn't see him again too soon!

As I came around from the procedure that day, I remember turning to the nurse in recovery and slurring, 'Is it over now? Please tell me it's actually over.'

'Yes,' she reassured me. 'You're all done now. You just need to rest.'

I'll be honest, I felt a kind of relief. Three full months of ups and downs in one treatment cycle had ended like this. The relief was palpable, but so was the emptiness.

Chapter 11

Time is a Healer

(and other myths)

THE EMPTINESS HUNG HEAVILY; I COULDN'T SHAKE IT. Cards and flowers from friends arrived (again). I felt like a person destined to live trapped in a perpetual cycle of everyone feeling sorry for them. I baulked at the thought of it. The sadness wore me down, it was thick and heavy above my head. It was as though the cloud that had begun to blow away over the past few years was back and I couldn't shake it.

I don't think you can compare grief; it simply isn't measurable and I think it's relative to what you have experienced in that moment and before. For me, this hurt *a lot*. I was grieving but not the same grief I had felt for Teddy. It was different, more confusing, even.

I hadn't looked pregnant, I hadn't been pregnant for a full nine months like I had with him but I had mapped out a potential future for this little one/s in the time we had gone through treatment and in all of the weeks of waiting afterwards. It felt as though the rug had been pulled out from under my feet; everything was gone, vanished. My body had been through so much trauma in such a short space of time and yet I felt guilty for grieving as, to the world, it appeared as though I had never even been pregnant.

The cycle of emptiness, guilt and confusion continued. My husband had planned to run a half marathon in London for Tommy's, the baby charity, the following week. We decided he would still do it. Now, more than ever, it felt important for us to be part of something positive and to support a charity that meant so much to us both. Their advice and support had been invaluable to me during these weeks of confusion and heartache losing this pregnancy. It felt comforting to know that I wasn't alone. I wasn't the only person who had lost a baby, or even lost a few. There were other parents out there just like us, navigating an impossibly complicated path. Raising money in Teddy's name was always important, no matter what was going on. It gave us both a way to feel like we were parenting him, in the only way we could.

So, just over a week after surgery, I went along to cheer. Seeing Nico run past filled me with pride as my eyes filled with tears. He would have been the best daddy – no, he *was* the best daddy. I still found it so difficult placing us in that narrative as Teddy's parents, without a child here to physically parent.

As the weeks went on, I hoped that time would be a healer. We were into April and a month away from Teddy's third birthday. So why was I still feeling worse than ever? I had been going for bi-weekly check-ups with my consultant to check that I was recovering. The blood test results on the day I had left the day surgery had shown my HCG was sky-high. No wonder I had felt so unwell. They had already sent all of the pregnancy for testing, in their words: 'To make sure there was nothing else going on, like a molar pregnancy.' I had read about those on the Tommy's website too. They seemed quite rare. Surely the chance of that on top of twins had to be slim to none? Initially, the test came back all clear, nothing to worry about.

On my next visit, my check-up was done by another consultant and my blood still contained a fairly high level of pregnancy hormone. A nurse that I had got to know well from the EPU came with me into the scan room so that the consultant could look at how I was healing and see if there was anything that might have been left.

'Things look normal,' he explained, 'but I can see a slight shadow. So, I'm not sure. We'll need to send everything to Charing Cross hospital to test it again, to check you don't have trophoblastic disease if it was a molar.'

Tropho-*what*?! He sounded so casual and I had no fucking idea what was going on at this point. I felt a wave of panic come over me. I had to have more bloods taken so, after I dressed, I was taken to my usual little room away from the waiting area. I felt like I should have had a plaque with my name on the door of that 'special room' by now. It was definitely where they took the continually unlucky to separate them from the throngs of pregnant bumps that lined the waiting corridor.

A few moments later, the kind nurse came back in, flanked by my usual consultant. Where had she sprung from so suddenly? The look on her face didn't give me the best vibes, to be honest. I had already been crying about the threat of another complication hanging over us, so I assumed she was just here to explain why there was yet more testing to go on.

'Your HCG is still high, you know that,' she said, as if to get me up to speed with it all. 'I have just taken a look at the images of your scan today and I'm not sure, I can't be 100 per cent sure, that it's all clear. Given your obstetric history, I need to be sure and I don't want to leave anything unchecked – you've been through enough. Which is why we are going to re-check with Charing Cross that we haven't missed anything, that it's not a possible molar pregnancy, and to rule out trophoblastic disease.' All of this I had heard before, so I nodded along. Then she added: 'That's a rare form of molar, a kind of uterine cancer.'

What the *fuck*? Had I just heard that correctly? I didn't say a word, for a few moments I didn't even move. Then, my hands rose to my face and I let out what sounded like a howl. The howl turned to sobs and I could barely see both her and the nurse though my tears. This was my breaking point. I couldn't take any more of this utter shitstorm.

'How can I be this unlucky? How could anyone be this unlucky? I had to be the first person who has ever embarked on IVF to have another baby and, three months later, was left not only having lost two babies but now potentially with cancer. Are you kidding me?'

My words were manic, barely comprehendible through the sobs and, by the looks on their faces, the answer was no, no one in that room was kidding me. The nurse squeezed me with a reassuring hug.

'You're right, no one should have to go through this. You've been so strong.'

I didn't feel strong, I felt desperate. My consultant sat beside me on the next chair as I took my face from my cupped hands. I looked at her, desperately wanting her to give me one shred of good news, anything right now that might help. She put her hand onto mine and looked at me, and then she said, 'I promise you that we'll get you through this and I promise you that before I retire, you'll have more babies. You'll have healthy babies, I promise, I'll make sure you do.'

She had no idea how much those words saved me just then. How she genuinely talked me down from the ledge that day. Maybe she didn't know that for sure – I mean, how *could* she? But it was what I needed to hear in that moment, in that room where I had felt the walls were closing in on me. It was the only hope I had to cling to, that there would be more babies in our future and that she was in our corner, doing everything she could to help us get there.

My head pounded as I left the hospital. How would I even begin to explain this one to everyone? I didn't want a pity-party, I was a one-woman-band where that was concerned anyway. I told my parents and a few close friends and then waited the next two weeks for results. I think I must have phoned the consultant's secretary at least a couple of times too, just to check on the off-chance that a result had come early. It was my birthday that week and I didn't want this hanging over us.

I tried to busy myself (I was a master at busying myself these days) with work or the garden. The house extension was well underway, so I was dealing with the builders, project managing it all (absolutely no clue what I was up to there) and trying to make decisions on what we wanted where and what dimensions things should be. Going through all of this while choosing taps, tiles and windows. However, it certainly helped take my mind off the wait. Two days before my birthday my phone rang, 'NO CALLER ID', and I knew it was my consultant. This was it.

'I'm going to put you out of your misery before I say anything else. It was all clear. No molar, no disease, nothing sinister.'

I felt like I exhaled properly, fully, for the first time in weeks.

'Thank you!' came tumbling out of my mouth straight away. 'This is the best birthday present.'

'I am concerned about your bloods though. They are dropping but you still have HCG and we need to take another look at that shadow we saw on the last scan. So we'll get you in for another scan in the next few weeks and then I think another hysteroscopy once you've had a period, just to see that we're not dealing with anything else in there.'

'Yes, absolutely. Anything you need to check again.' I was on cloud nine. I didn't have anything serious to worry about, they could check what they liked. For months, the past few years even, my only concern had been getting pregnant again but these two weeks had put a lot into perspective for me. It wasn't just about having another baby or not – this had become about my health, about a risk to my own health. It had all been born out of a need for another baby, to jump back on the treatment merry-go-round and try again each month. I realised I didn't want to do that again just now. I was happy for her to check things out, have another look around in there, but I needed a break. My body needed a break, *we* needed a break from this.

The guilt hung as heavily as the emptiness did. Now, finally, I really did think I needed to '*talk to someone*'. It was a question that I was asked so much after Teddy died: 'Are you talking to someone?' – the emphasis always flung heavily on the final word. 'Someone' being a person in a professional capacity, be it a counsellor, therapist or a psychologist. A firm 'No' had always been my answer. I hadn't wanted to talk to anyone outside of our family and close friends – why would I? They didn't know me, they couldn't understand, unless of course the exact same succession of tragic events had happened to them.

Except now I began to feel differently. Though I was conflicted about who I might speak to and what benefit I might gain from it. I debated in my head the pros and cons of opening up to a stranger about the past month's events. The pros seemed to outweigh anything else and I was tired of feeling like a burden on my family. I had grown weary of my own sadness and felt guilty that its complexities were beginning to weigh heavily on the people I loved the most too. So, as a 34th birthday treat to myself, I decided to get myself Helen.

It was entirely by accident as I had stumbled across Helen's business card as I sat in the waiting room for my acupuncture appointment one day. It was during the week of the 'You might have a rare kind of cancer' chat and my head was full of what-ifs and a general sense of confusion. As I looked up from my phone to the coffee table in front of me, there was a pile of Helen's cards staring me in the face. I hastily bundled one into my bag and then proceeded to walk around with it on my person for at least a week before I felt confident enough to actually call her. Her voice was soft and welcoming; she sounded as though she had a calming energy (exactly the kind I needed right now).

My first meeting with her was about 90 minutes long. I had to explain the whole sorry tale of how I had come to be sitting in the chair in front of her. It wasn't a short story and I only realised when speaking to someone completely new that I struggled to say some parts of the story aloud, or even let my mind walk back through those moments. She let me pause when I needed, offered tissues at the appropriate moments and just allowed me to spill my innermost thoughts and feelings out into that tiny room. People were *right,* it *was* good to talk. It was agreed I would see her every other week, safe in the sanctuary of the comfy arm-chair of that room. We began, bit by bit, to unpick the events of the last three years and my emotions around trying again for another baby. And so my journey into therapy began.

I enjoyed turning 34 that weekend more than I could have imagined. No, I wasn't pregnant but I wasn't un-well either. I was ready to give myself a few months off, at least. I just wanted to relax and enjoy life, just a bit, for a while. Just while we picked ourselves up from this. No more drugs, or Chinese herbs, or weird shit. A total break. Which felt quite liberating at this point.

Before I knew it, we were heading to Cornwall again and staring down the barrel of Teddy's third birthday. Three. How were we here already? In some ways, it had gone in the blink of an eye, yet in others it felt as though we were a million miles away from that day three years ago. Everything, and yet nothing, had changed. I had pictured us by now bringing Teddy's little brother or sister down to Cornwall with us. Sitting on his beach together and writing his name in the sand. Yet it was still just us, the three amigos: me, Nico and Boris (the pug). The weather was stunning and for that I was so grateful; I needed everything I could get to boost my mood. I'd had so much to worry about, medically, that I hadn't allowed myself to give Teddy's birthday a second thought. Then, without warning, the enormity of three whole years without him hit me like a tidal wave.

I woke on the morning of his birthday with an instant heaviness hanging over my head. I hadn't been expecting it. I had thought after his first birthday that each year would get easier, the weight a little lighter, and that had felt true the previous year. But today felt very different. A *three-year-old* was missing, not a baby. I couldn't shake that feeling of emptiness, from losing Teddy to the recent months of confusion and loss. It all suddenly felt too heavy to take anymore. I remember sitting on the floor of the kitchen and sobbing, big heavy tears that wouldn't fade, that didn't get any lighter. My heart hurt again, like it did in those early days of grief.

I think it was that day, possibly the first day ever in those three years, that I started to lose sight of hope. The hope that there would be better days coming, more children in our future, was what had kept me going. I could see that hope slipping through my fingers and I couldn't seem to catch hold of it. In the days that followed I said to my husband, 'What if we never get to do it again, be parents? What if I never get the privilege to carry another baby, what if I can't? What if it's just us, forever?' Forever was starting to feel like an awfully long time. He put his arm around my shoulders as we both sat on the beach, early in the morning, to mark three years since Teddy left us, and he said:

'Well, if it's just us, then that's not so bad, is it?'

He was right, it wasn't, but I was scared.

'We'll find a way, I promise,' he finished.

Those two weeks away were what I needed to help process the intense grief I was feeling for what we had just been through. It allowed me to sit with it and acknowledge it and not to try to rush through it and 'feel better' like I had done at the start of 2017. It also gave me a chance to think about the months ahead, about *not* pursuing any more treatment, for now.

When we returned home it was easy to not think about it, as we were in the final weeks of our house project and there was *so* much to be done. So, I spent the rest of May and June painting, organising and trying to get everything finished so we could move back into that end of the house. We'd spent the past four months with no running water downstairs or anywhere to wash our clothes; I was looking forward to saying goodbye to launderette trips and washing up dishes in the bath! The final furlong of the project seemed to go on for years instead of weeks but it gave me the distraction, after everything, that I needed.

I had the pleasure of my next hysteroscopy on the first day of July. Planned around my cycle, it was in my calendar ready to be performed at exactly the right time. It would happen before my next review and planning meeting at the IVF clinic, so we would know exactly what we were dealing with. I went in on a Monday morning, assured by my consultant that she had booked me in with their top guy for the job. She made him sound like the best in the business; if anyone could find something that was upsetting the feng shui in there, then it was him. Having had the procedure before (and a lot worse in recent months), I didn't feel unduly worried this time. I felt calm, if anything. I just wanted to know what was happening in there.

I went into the same room in which I'd had the same procedure more than two years previously. I changed in the cubicle into my gown, ready for action, and the next thing I knew I was up on the bed with my legs in stirrups and the brightest of lights shining between my thighs. It brought an entirely new meaning to the phrase 'being in the spotlight'. The doctor was an older man, polite and direct – very direct. He peered at me over his spectacles and down to my medical notes as he double-checked my name.

'So, the reason we are doing this today, on recommendation from your doctor, is just to take a look around in your uterus and double-check there is nothing that has been missed on scans. No retained products of pregnancy, no scarring, nothing that shouldn't be in there. OK? Let's get started.'

Just like that, it was underway with no further warning. *Fuuuuuuuck!* (Inner dialogue, you'll be relieved to hear.) That was quicker and more painful than I remembered; I am pretty sure I almost broke the nurse's hand. What, hang on?! Was it over?

As he emerged from between my knees, he swivelled almost immediately on his chair back around to my notes on a desk, where he began scribbling things down while tapping at his computer keys simultaneously. The nurses all remained silent, as if they knew to wait for him to speak. I still lay there, knees knocking, scarred from the brutality and speed of the experience.

'Well, yes,' he began. 'It looks as though you still have some debris in there that will need clearing. Which your consultant will arrange. Although I am not entirely sure how recent it is? Perhaps still there from your previous loss?'

Debris, that needed *clearing*. He sounded as if he were sorting out a minor incident on the M25 not informing me of the inner workings of my uterus. What a way to break the news.

I was barely taking in his words and mustering my reply when he said: 'Right, so if you want to get yourself up and dressed. Thank you and have a good day.' The nurses were already hastily ushering me up and off the bed and removing paper coverings to replace with fresh ones for her next patient.

'So, will I hear . . .' I began nervously, not wanting to inconvenience him.

'You'll hear from your consultant again soon; she'll take it from here. Thank you.'

He still didn't look up from his keypad or notes, his back still turned. I got the feeling that his thank you was a polite, *Please fuck off now, I'm busy and a have about a hundred more complicated vaginas to inspect today.*

Blimey, that *was* direct. But by Friday that week I had a call from my consultant:

'There's definitely something in there. I'm looking at the pictures from your hysteroscopy now. Could be scarring? It's in a top corner, almost around the corner, out of sight, which will be why we've never found it. We need to get you in to remove it and I want to do that quickly, before you have an IVF plan in place. We need to get this sorted for you.'

Before I could answer, she continued: 'I have a space for you next week, on Thursday. We can operate then and then this should be over for you.'

It sounded so full and final. Was whatever had been hanging around in there the culprit to all of these problems, all along? How long had it been 'just out of sight'? I had so many questions but I knew she couldn't answer them now. The only way she would know more was if I agreed to the op next week, which of course, I did.

I couldn't comprehend how I could possibly be going in for another operation. It seemed like madness but I wanted this sorted and I trusted that it was in my best interests. Perhaps it would change the outcome of any future IVF treatment for us? Perhaps whatever was in there was what had caused my missed miscarriage? I was coming to learn that with secondary infertility and the treatment we had undergone since, there were always going to be questions whirring around my head, most of them remaining unanswered.

I was back in the anaesthetic room that very next week. Same jokes, same cold tingle up my arm. I had started to play a weird game with myself each time I went under, to see how long I could resist and stay awake before it got me (probably not one I would or should recommend but it kept me entertained). The positive to come out of all of this was that after five sedations in five months, I had more or less conquered my fear of it. Like I say, small wins, hey?

I awoke to the sight of a friendly nurse and the groaning of a woman in the next bay to me in the recovery room. I was weary and in pain, I remember feeling sick this time as I woke. As I lay there, the pain gradually got worse. I asked for more pain relief, something I don't think I'd ever done after any of the procedures there. What had they done? The cramping was intense but the morphine certainly helped to take the edge off.

They wheeled me back to the ward and my consultant greeted me – she was smiling. If she looked pleased then I certainly felt it. I waited with bated breath and she began to speak:

'I'm really happy with how it went. I am confident we got everything. It was tricky and it took time, but we got there.'

A rush of something came over me. Hope, maybe? After all of this, all this time and tears, it felt like it was finally, *really*, over.

Chapter 12

Round Three . . .

THE REST OF JULY PASSED WITHOUT SO MUCH AS A TRIP TO THE HOSPITAL. It felt like a big change, a relief. It was somewhere that I had become so used to spending so many hours of my life, waiting for appointments or blood tests, being wheeled around corridors between procedures. A break was welcome. I was healing well after my last operation and, although I was a little weary from the last few months' goings-on, it was nice to think that things might be a little more straightforward from here on in. That my encounters with the dildo wand might become less frequent and that there would (hopefully) be less chat about debris/scarring/

whatever the hell had been hanging around in there for the past months.

It had also been over five months since our last IVF round had come to an end and more than four since the weeks of waiting and operations that unravelled thereafter. My body had enjoyed a break from the hormones that had caused a sense of constant turmoil. I was beginning to feel like I was in a place where I might consider doing it all again.

I was realistic about time. I knew that any new cycle would take up two months of the year at the very least. If it were to become a successful treatment cycle, resulting in a pregnancy, then it would be another eight weeks on top of that before we were at the point of having a 12-week scan. I knew those first weeks of pregnancy would be filled with nothing but fear and uncertainty for me, especially given our most recent experience. I didn't want to enter into this with a blinkered idea of how it might feel or how intense that four-month timeframe might be. We needed to be sure that we were ready to go through it all again, this side of Christmas. Yes, it was early August and I was already considering Christmas again. Déjà vu? The months and cycles were stealing our years, with two, three, four months at a time flying by.

I had my check-up with my consultant who seemed happy that my lining was thick enough to indicate that a period would be any day. My hormone levels were as would be expected too, nothing there that shouldn't be. She was, of course, right. My period arrived in a timely fashion, just in time for our next review appointment at the IVF clinic. We had last walked out of there in early March, grasping a report that had told us our baby had miscarried. Five months later, we were walking back in eager to hear how we might push forward in our pursuit to become parents again.

I wasn't sure now how I felt about those photos of smiling babies that adorned the walls of the waiting areas and stairwell. At first, I had found them so hopeful but they had started to become a symbol of everything we had yet to achieve. I could see why they were there. I knew that if our treatment was to ever be a success and we had another baby that I would almost certainly be the mum who sent in a photo of my beautiful miracle.

The review went well and it was agreed that we could start again, although a few of my screenings needed to be updated (cervical and STDs) which could easily be solved by a quick appointment with the nurse at the GP surgery. The IVF consultant thought it a good idea for us to pursue another fresh round, meaning another round of stimulation and egg retrieval. The last round had given us just three day-five embryos: one had been transferred, one other was good enough to freeze, the third embryo had not made the cut. I couldn't help but feel another little wave of sadness wash over me in the moment when I learned that the third embryo had not made it to freezing. It felt so callous that, after all of those efforts, it could just be discarded and considered 'not good enough'. I do recall asking that we be informed at the time if that were to happen again – not so much to influence the decision either way but just so we knew what was going to happen and why. Having just one embryo on ice meant that pursuing a frozen round of treatment could be considered a bit of a risky business: essentially, what if we got to the point where we were ready for transfer and that one little chance didn't survive the thawing process? It would mean that six weeks of treatment would have been for nothing. We knew we weren't emotionally capable of taking that risk at this point, and we still had options.

Although, the thought of another fresh round also felt intimidating. The entire process from start to finish felt so long. It was in that moment that I understood why so many couples must just say 'enough now, no more'. It feels quite daunting each time the prospect of more treatment is mapped out in front of you. When you're handed that piece of paper with drugs and dates listed on it. For some, it's just too much to bear, I would imagine. We weren't there yet though, we were ready to give it another crack. For us, that next crack of the whip looked like it would start in a couple of weeks, on day 21 of this very cycle. I felt a mix of excitement and nerves. I couldn't face the same thing happening again; it *had* to be better this time.

I was scheduled to go back in just two weeks' time, providing they had the latest report from my consultant on the success of my recent procedure and all of my screenings were up to date. I just had to get hold of all of the relevant paperwork to support that and then we would be good to go. (In)fertility admin should have an entire section of this book dedicated to it, really. I don't feel like I am doing it justice. The time, the phone calls, the letters, the tests, the scanning and sending of paperwork; more tests, the chasing of results ... It is endless, relentless. Working from home, I found ways to make it manageable and tried my best not to let it take over my days but I had friends who were teachers, civil servants, midwives and they had to try to cram all of this in around demanding work, even delivering other people's babies. It seemed an impossible amount of life-admin sometimes. I wondered how many hours I had already clocked up just driving to and from the fertility clinic? Much, much longer than the 20-minute fumble that it must take some couples to conceive when they 'weren't even trying'! I am aware that sounds incredibly bitter, but I promise I am just poking fun (no innuendo intended either!). I spent those two weeks committing to that last little bit of (in)fertility admin, desperately trying to get those metaphorical ducks in a row so we could get the green light.

On the morning of my next appointment, I arrived alone, a bag full of the relevant paperwork and eager to collect my first assortment of needles and drugs. I was ready to seamlessly cartwheel back onto the baby making merry-go-round and hoping this time things would work out differently. The appointment consisted (again) of checking and double-checking everything. An extended box-ticking exercise. Luckily, Nico had fulfilled all of his requirements on this front upon our last meeting with the consultant so I was free to fly solo this time. I was starting to shoulder the guilt of how much time he had had to take out from his busy job and I knew he was beginning to feel like he wasn't

committing to either properly. He was stretching him-
self between trying to support us through this and trying to do his best at work. I wanted him to be able to
be there, for this, when he absolutely needed to be and
otherwise I would happily go alone. That felt like less
stress and pressure for us, although I know it would be
different for everyone.

Before they let me down to the pharmacy, I was also
taken through the injections again. How to administer
each one, the drugs I would be using and what each
did. I was set to embark on two weeks of my very best
friend again, buserelin, and I hoped (oh, how I hoped)
that taking it during the warmer and lighter months
would turn me into less of a moody bitch . . .! I would
then be back for a baseline scan before they began me
on stimulation drugs again, to get those follicles going.
That would be at the end of the first week of September. We were set to go to Cornwall after that appointment to try to catch a little bit of the late-summer sunshine. I was very much aiming for the 'relax and enjoy'
frame of mind for this treatment round. Last time, I
had been too caught up in the yoga and meditation,
the Chinese herbs and acupuncture. This time, I really
wanted to go with the flow and try to allow my body
just to do its thing.

The buserelin wasn't as bad as I recalled. I got the odd headache but nothing bad this time. I found myself fitting it into my everyday life a lot better too. I was stressing less about having to be at home when it was injection time in the evening and was injecting in the car before meeting friends, in restaurant toilets – basically anywhere I had to in order to carry on with normal life. Before I had let it dictate everything, but not this time. This time felt different, like I was an old hand now. This was just what I had to do if we were going to make it through the next few weeks successfully.

My baseline scan went without a hitch. Everything was behaving itself in there. My ovaries were suitably quiet and my lining was thin. Check! I collected my stimulation drugs and we set off to Cornwall that same day. I hadn't told anyone (apart from my mum) we were doing treatment this time; it felt better that way. The stress of having to explain the ups and downs of the last loss had really taken its toll – I couldn't explain why we were embarking on this again to more people.

By some stroke of a miracle, the sun shone in Cornwall for the entire week! The beaches were quiet, our walks were long and the sunsets were stunning. I didn't feel like I was doing treatment at all; it was the polar opposite to last time. Obviously, there were the standard no-gos with treatment and I couldn't enjoy the pleasure of a G&T while we watched those picture-perfect sunsets, but it didn't matter. It felt easier somehow and I felt content instead of worried about every little thing. I was certain that this would be doing my body some good (especially the vitamin D from that beautiful sunshine!).

The week went by in a flash and, before I knew it, I was back at the clinic. Lying on the bed in the scanning room. Pen and Post-It note in hand, ready to write down those all-important scores on the ovarian boards. Those little follies didn't let me down either. It seems that they had equally enjoyed their week of sunshine and relaxation and everything seemed to be doing (and most importantly growing!) well. I had a lot of follicles this time and my body was having a far more positive response than it had done before. *Great news*, I thought to myself. *Maybe we'll get more than three embryos?* More embryos, more chances, right?

Before I went to the pharmacy I saw another nurse who updated me on the progress so far and explained that they would keep a close eye on everything in my next tracking appointment, as things could also go *too* well and they didn't want me to end up being at risk of OHSS (ovarian hyper-stimulation syndrome).

OHSS would mean my ovaries going into overdrive and producing too many follicles, which puts your health at risk, and embryo transfer wouldn't happen in most cases as the risks are too high. We were back walking that tightrope, keeping a fine balance, this time battling things going *too* well.

I went straight into London for an appointment with Emma later that morning. I had decided to book two sessions with her for this cycle as I wanted to try to increase my chances of good stimulation first and then see her again after transfer. She helped to calm me down when I explained that my ovaries had changed their mind and decided to put in an over-time shift for this round. She explained to me about the unpredictability of fertility treatment and how we must try to relinquish that control in our mind and our body if it was to be a success. She reminded me not to put too much pressure on myself and to trust in the process. She was right of course, as she had been all along. I allowed myself to relax in that session and tried to visualise everything growing at a slow and steady pace. I came away feeling less like things were spiralling out of control again.

Two days later, I was back at the clinic for an update. It seemed so strange how I had gone from willing my follicles to grow to now willing them to slow the fuck down! They still seemed to be going full steam ahead. The nurse spoke to the consultant who advised to cut my dosage right down. This was in the hope that they could slow down the ones that were maturing quickly and the rest would just get to the right size for egg retrieval at the beginning of next week. I couldn't imagine that we would be delaying that procedure in this round – quite the opposite. I also felt physically different this time. I was bloated and my tummy was beginning to feel tight, almost like the beginning of a pregnancy when everything starts to stretch and grow. I was also *really* thirsty, much more so than these drugs had ever made me before.

When my final scan rolled around at the end of the week, it was confirmed we were more than ready to go to egg retrieval on Monday. I had 42 follicles. A number that would have seemed an impossible amount in my last treatment round. They told me that not all of these would be big enough to release a mature egg and that I was at high-risk of OHSS. I had already begun to hear the words 'freeze all' banded around in appointments. This means a round where embryos are created but nothing is transferred back in, as the risk of becoming severely poorly with OHSS would be too great. Of course, I knew this wouldn't happen to me, it rarely happened and only *ever* when they collected more than 25 mature eggs. I was hardly going to go from zero, to ten, to *more* than twenty-five, was I? It seemed an impossibility . . .

I was on the lowest dose of stimulation drug for those last injections and administered that final trigger shot over the weekend. I rested, drank more water than you could imagine was possible and even fitted in a pub lunch with friends. I remember feeling like a fraud as I sat there in my baggy dress and tights, feeling as though I was about to burst but not daring to tell anyone why I felt so awful. Instead, I sipped on my water and plastered on a smile. I had become a master in the art of this by now.

The next morning at 7am we were back in the waiting room of the day surgery unit with that sea of faces sitting around us, also waiting for their fate to be decided. It was much quieter than last time and I felt like the whole process was quicker. Everything seems to become easier when you know what lies ahead. The check-in, the check lists, the surgical stockings, the banter with the nurses about 'the sample room'. We chatted and waited, and watched *Good Morning Britain* as the collapse of Thomas Cook unravelled on the television screen in front of our eyes. We knew what we were doing and it felt happy and relaxed this time. My main worry was still how many eggs they were set to retrieve that day. I was worried it would all be over in there. The bloating I'd experienced over the weekend was to be expected as my ovaries were swollen by this point. But I had been told it could get much worse after retrieval as that's when the fluid from all of those follicles begins to escape out into your body.

It must have been playing on my mind a lot as, much like last time, my first question on waking up was 'How many did they get?' followed swiftly by 'Please tell me it wasn't more than 25?' And, just like last time, I was told that the embryologist would be the one to deliver that news when I was out of recovery and back in my room. I was itching to get out of that recovery room but I also couldn't ignore the fact that I was already beginning to feel the size of a barrage balloon, swollen and tight.

They wheeled me back in and I felt groggy as hell. Nico was sitting there, a bag of snacks on my tray table at the ready. It was a few minutes before the embryologist came to see us. It was a different lady to last time, perhaps my age (I wish, definitely younger) and quite possibly one of the cheeriest people I had ever met. I decided you definitely have to be cheery when you work in embryology, when you might have to deliver news that was so important to people. I felt increasingly sick as we began to listen.

'OK,' she began. 'So, we successfully retrieved 28 mature eggs. Which, as you know, means we'll have to speak with the consultant but it looks as though re-gardless of how many embryos do well over these next days that we'll be heading for a freeze-all cycle.'

Twenty-fucking-eight.

Freeze-fucking-all.

Fuck.

Chapter 13

Oh(ss)

For F*ck's Sake

I PASTED ON A SMILE, AND THEN BROKE INTO SOBS THE MOMENT SHE LEFT THE ROOM.

'Well, that's that then,' I wept to my husband as I held my hands to cover my face. He rubbed my arm and tried his best to soothe me as I shook with tears. It all seemed, at one point, as though it had been going so well. *Too* well, you might say. Now this, an abundance of eggs, and yet no matter how many embryos we achieved this time absolutely everything would be going on ice, until we were able to pursue another round in the future. And right now that felt like light years away.

The rubbing on my arm was starting to make me feel sick, really sick actually. The room looked a little hazy as it began to spin. The last thing I remember at that point was declaring that I desperately needed a wee, before waking up in a crumpled heap on the floor next to the base of my drip stand. Luckily, Nico had jumped up and caught me on the way down just as a nurse had been entering the room to come and check on us. They helped me back into bed and the nurse explained that they would need to keep me on a drip for the rest of the day and start me on some anti-sickness medication. This was the start of OHSS, I knew it was. Everything felt different from the last time I had woken up from this procedure. My head was pounding, I felt like I couldn't take in enough air when I drew breath and when I looked down at my tummy, it was already beginning to look swollen and distended. Last time, in comparison to this, I had practically skipped out of there.

We spent the rest of the day in hospital. It wasn't until the early evening that I hobbled back to the car supported by my husband. Every bump on the car journey home made me want to vomit; I felt sore from head to toe. It was all I could do to shower and crawl into bed when we returned, Boris curled at my side, my ever-faithful furry friend always ready when I needed him.

When I woke the next morning, I knew we would be expecting a phone call from the embryologists. Regardless of what the plan was, they needed to update us on how many of those eggs had fertilised and how many embryos we had. The call came in, the same lovely lady from yesterday, first of all checking on how I was feeling. I couldn't help but notice how genuinely concerned she sounded when she asked me, too, as if it wasn't just protocol but that she knew I must be feeling beyond disappointed at the prospect of no transfer. Not to mention the physical pain of the fluid that was currently making its way into my uterus and beyond. I had woken up with a new barrel-shaped abdomen and the tightness was almost unbearable. She explained that a nurse would be calling to check on me later today too and that I would need to go back to the hospital tomorrow for a scan and check-up. She then proceeded to break the news we were really interested in . . .

Twenty-three eggs had fertilised. I was in shock. Suddenly my thoughts of despair turned into tears of elation as I pictured that whole rugby team (and reserves bench) of embryos waiting in the lab for us. I knew they would all be going on ice but this number felt too good to be true. I couldn't wait to tell Nico, who was over the moon too. Then I called my mum.

Bad news had become good and I was grasping for all of the positives I could find right now because I felt bloody awful still. Like I might pop, actually.

The following day, we drove to the hospital to get checked up. Just as well, as I had swollen to the size of a small village. I had been on a drug called cabergoline to help with the fluid and some anti-sickness medication to counteract its effects, plus the usual progesterone pessaries. It's fair to say that the concoction was making me feel pretty rotten by this point. I could barely sit as we waited to be taken through. Even wearing clothes was making me feel sick. I stood and sipped water.

The scan showed over a litre and a half of fluid in my uterus. It had begun to 'seep out', as she put it, and was starting to surround my other organs. No wonder I felt like shit. They needed to treat it as soon as possible. The remaining hope of any embryo transfer was completely out of the equation now and, to be honest, the idea of any more poking or prodding, let alone the prospect of pregnancy hormones being thrown into the mix, made me want to run a mile (more of a slow, gasping waddle right now). They made the decision to take me off progesterone, as I wouldn't need it with no transfer happening, and put me back on buserelin injections until my period showed up. I would keep on taking the cabergoline, rest and drink water. I couldn't do much else right now anyway; walking was enough of a struggle.

I was gutted to be back on the buserelin injections already. I had only bid goodbye to my marathon of injections just five days ago with that final trigger shot and had felt so smug about it too! Still, at least I knew where I was with this drug, it was nothing new, and if it made me feel even a fraction better then I was all for it right now. I stayed in bed for the next 48 hours, sleeping, flicking through magazines and drinking as many fluids as I could. The swelling just seemed to stay there but the nurses assured me that it would sub-side quickly as soon as my period came. So, naturally, I spent most of my time willing for that to make an early appearance.

We had also made it to day five with our embryos and had another 13 to add to the bank. They would go on ice, for now, but I took great comfort in the fact that they would be joining our one little lone ranger from the last round. It sounds so strange to say but I felt as though it wouldn't be lonely anymore with 13 new friends for company. Yes, I had given my embryos feelings.

With the embryos firmly in the freezer and our dreams also on ice, the only thing to focus on was feeling better. That weekend was another of bed rest while I awaited my period. I hobbled down into town on the Monday morning to see my regular acupuncturist and hope that she could help me. It was the furthest I had walked in a week – actually, the only place I had walked in a week. By the time I arrived, I was breathless and flustered and she looked a little shocked at the sight of me. I remember asking if there was any way she could just stick a needle in and pop me like a balloon. That felt like a reasonable request right now.

The acupuncture, the buserelin and the other drugs seemed to do the trick and within a few days I practically screamed with delight when my period arrived. As promised by the nurses, the relief and change in my body was almost instantaneous. By the following morning I looked distinctly less swollen, I could bend, breathe and when I laughed it didn't hurt. I called the clinic to let them know. They said I could stop all drugs and leave things to settle down naturally now.

At the check-up scan a week later, I was given the all clear. OHSS had been crazy, it seemed to appear out of nowhere, cause a world of pain and then simply disappear as swiftly as it had arrived, leaving no trace. I think this was when it really began to set in, the disappointment of how this round had ended. When I had still been feeling so unwell I had felt vaguely relieved, but now I felt better again physically, it just gave me the time and space to think about what could have been. We should have been firmly in the midst of a two-week wait again but we were on hold once more.

When I went in to see the nurse after my scan I cried on her. I explained how I was beginning to feel hopeless at this whole process all over again and how I was so confused by how my body had reacted so differently with each round of treatment. I told her all about Teddy and how we longed to be parents again. Luckily for me, I struck gold with the most understanding nurse I could have hoped for. She had just returned to work herself from maternity leave.

'I do understand how you feel, I really do.' Something in the way she spoke told me she truly did. She went on to tell me about her own battle with secondary infertility, about losing her own baby who had been stillborn and about her multiple rounds of IVF and miscarriages. She *did* get it. She told me that she had just returned to work after having her son, who was conceived naturally.

'I know you feel so desperate in this moment, but I promise you, you will get there.'

She held my hand and I knew she was feeling every inch of my pain and emptiness as I sat and poured my heart out. I told her how I needed to start again, to feel like we were moving forward, not sitting still and waiting. I begged her to ask the consultant to look at options, that I was willing to try anything. I watched as she considered her response and I could see she wanted to help me.

It was agreed by the consultant that, as I had had a period to end that last cycle and we had so many embryos on ice, he would allow, just this once, letting us try a natural cycle. This wasn't something our clinic usually offered as it was considered less controlled (for obvious reasons, as you are entirely at the mercy of the body doing its own thing naturally, which, let's face it, mine wasn't renowned for). She broke it down for me: as I was at the start of my cycle already, they could give me some progress scans the following week to check my lining and, if everything looked good and I ovulated naturally, then they would thaw and transfer an embryo at the time that conception would occur naturally. Then I would be given progesterone to try to support a pregnancy. It sounded *so* simple. A new way of trying.

It seemed like the perfect solution, worth a gamble, and worth not having to take medication for. I wasn't sure if my body really knew what was going on after the OHSS but perhaps we could trick it into doing the right thing? I had to go straight back in the next day for a booking appointment that had been scheduled at the last minute. This round of treatment involved another set of paperwork to be filled out, for my husband to give his permission (again) for one of the banked embryos to be transferred.

The hope and potential of this new treatment idea turned out to be short-lived for us. I was just two scans in when it was deemed I would have inadequate lining and likely wouldn't ovulate that month. *There go those ovaries shutting up shop again*, I thought. Probably pissed at me that we put them to work for 28 eggs last cycle and so had perhaps decided that would be their last contribution for a while. It turned out that it wasn't just the embryos I was giving thoughts and feelings to!

I felt crestfallen but not surprised that this too-good-to-be-true treatment plan hadn't miraculously worked for us first time. I knew that the nurse had just been doing her best to find a way for us, *any* way. I'd allowed myself to get swept up in the hope and the what-ifs that it might be the right thing to do, straight away, without any gaps between cycles. As I cried on yet another nurse that day it was agreed I would see the consultant again the following month for a proper review of everything. November. We had made it to November, nearing the end of *another* year. I couldn't believe it.

The next few weeks hurtled by as they always seemed to at that time of year and the evenings drew in. My OHSS from the beginning of the previous month was already feeling like a distant memory, one I would most definitely rather forget. As we sat in his office that day, I seemed to get a sense from the consultant that he was genuinely sorry, not to mentioned a little baffled, at how differently each of our cycles had turned out so far. A cancellation due to poor response, a success resulting in twin miscarriage and now, a freeze-all and a bout of OHSS.

'With each cycle we learn something new,' he began, 'but, sometimes, the body can be somewhat unpredictable. So, if we were to ever do another fresh cycle, which thankfully I don't think we need to, given how many chances we have on ice, I would be hard pushed to predict which way it would go again next time.'

I felt like a medical phenomenon, and not in a good way.

'I think what we can safely say is that we will need to do another medicated cycle but that would be a frozen cycle, using one of the embryos we already have. We can start that as soon as you have your next period, so you must call us when that happens. Although it's been really upsetting for you both, I want you to remain positive as you have 14 frozen embryos: that's a lot of chances before we have to explore our next options.'

So we would go around again, one more time. Except this time was a frozen round, another new experience for us. I was due my period in the next couple of weeks. When that happened I would call the clinic and we would get started. By my calculations, I wouldn't be starting medication until towards the end of December. Wonderful, *festive* injections! I couldn't stop thinking about what he said, though. He was right, we had 14 little chances in there.

Fourteen rays of hope, just waiting.

Chapter 14

In This Together

ONE OF THE FEELINGS THAT OFTEN OVERWHELMED ME ON THIS BUMPY ROAD OF LOSS AND FERTILITY WAS LONELINESS. It's easy to begin to feel isolated if no one in your immediate circle has ever experienced something similar to the road you are travelling. I have found so much comfort in connecting with other women online, through Instagram, blogs, podcasts and over emails exchanged. Hearing other people talk about their experiences has often shone a light for me when the road ahead looked too dark to travel.

I'll be forever grateful for the wonderful loss and TTC (Trying To Conceive) community online for keeping me going and for their willingness to share so openly about their journeys. I am aware that my personal story of loss and fertility struggles won't resonate with everyone and I don't aim to or expect to represent everyone. All of our struggles will be different – and our outcomes often differ too. I really hope that by including stories from other women in this chapter, together we will have helped more people to feel seen, heard and included in the conversation around fertility treatment and loss. I feel so honoured that these four brilliant women have been willing to be a part of this book and share their stories. So, I'll be quiet now and let them take it from here . . .

Life Before You
by Sophie Smith

I never thought I would get to write about our own happy ending. Our journey of trying to conceive our baby lasted six years and took a slightly different route to what we ever expected it to. It is definitely one that we will never forget.

Jack and I are true childhood sweethearts; we met at school when he was 16 and I was 14. We grew up together and got engaged in our mid-twenties before marrying three years later in 2012. Both of us always knew we wanted children but we also wanted to travel as much as we could before trying, so we waited another couple of years until we felt completely ready. At this point we didn't put ourselves under any pressure and tried to stay relaxed each month. Seven months later we got our first positive pregnancy test. We were both emotional and over the moon. We told our closest friends and family and we were totally ready for our lives to change.

At around seven weeks pregnant, I started having an excruciating pain in my side which lasted a few hours. A few days later, my symptoms disappeared and I had a feeling that something wasn't right. Just after Christmas, we decided to go for a private early scan to check everything. Coincidentally, on the morning of the scan, one of my best friends, Em, who I have known since we were 13, called to tell me she had just found out that she was also pregnant, meaning we would be only a few weeks apart. We were really excited to start this journey together.

Jack and I went into the scan room and the sonographer started examining me. Quite a bit of time passed and the room was silent. 'I think you need to go straight to A&E.' The scan had showed an ectopic pregnancy in my left fallopian tube. I vaguely knew what this meant but Jack didn't. As we left the clinic,

I vividly remember looking at his face as I explained to him what an ectopic pregnancy was and seeing his pain. That moment is something I'll never forget. I always thought that our first pregnancy would be magical and exciting. Unfortunately, we would never get that moment back again.

The medication I was given by the hospital to 'expel' the pregnancy didn't work and a week later I had surgery to remove my left tube.

A few months later, we were lucky enough to get pregnant again but at six and a half weeks I started bleeding. This was our second loss in a short space of time. After that, we went to a private doctor and tests showed we needed to go straight for IVF treatment because I only had one fallopian tube and a low AMH (egg reserve), so it was felt our time to conceive was limited.

It was a year after our second loss that we started our first IVF treatment. We transferred two embryos and had a positive test ten days later. An early scan gave us some hope, showing a sac and foetal pole, but a week later it was again confirmed that the pregnancy had stopped developing at seven weeks. Unfortunately, the medication that I was given didn't work again and a few weeks later I miscarried while on holiday. Three losses down and the grief started to set in.

We were now three years into our journey and about to start our next round of IVF but it wasn't going to be simple. Just before we started the round, we had two very early pregnancy losses over consecutive months. These became losses four and five.

The grief started to eat away at me and I could feel myself changing as a person. I felt embarrassed and lost. It became increasingly hard as many of my friends started to have babies and I felt overwhelmed with envy. I had a permanent lump in my throat and felt in so much pain, and then the guilt about feeling this way would set in and the vicious circle continued. The ache for our own baby was so great that my anxiety rose each day. Why not me?

I could only rely on Jack to know exactly how I was feeling but there were days when even he couldn't help me. Grieving for lost pregnancies, with the hormones and mixed emotions inside me, created such desperation. I spent a fortune on acupuncture, herbs and reflexology to try to do whatever I could to help.

After a bit of a break and another year later, we got pregnant again through IVF at a new clinic. But once again the pregnancy didn't last longer than seven weeks. This was loss number six, although by this point we had nearly lost count. The emotional pain was immense and I was so desperate for it all to be over. I wanted to experience all the little things I was watching others around me do with their babies – buying Christmas pyjamas, going for baby swimming lessons and sensory classes, giving them their first foods or watching their first steps.

It was at this point that I felt at my lowest. I couldn't go into work (I had a highly pressured job as a buyer) and dreaming of having a baby took over my every thought. I was very lucky to have incredible family and friends around me who I could lean on and I will forever feel grateful that they were there.

One day, in the midst of this time, Em came over to see us. She told me that, if it came to it, she would like to help us have a baby and be our surrogate. I didn't take it all in at the time and, although I thought it was the kindest offer, I really didn't think she was being serious. A couple of weeks later we received an email from Em and her husband James that documented the seriousness of their offer and it was only then that we started to believe them. We had never considered surrogacy and I was still in a place where I wanted to try to carry our own child, but the fact that there was another option gave us back some hope. If we were to ever decide surrogacy was our best option then I knew I trusted Em implicitly to be the woman who helped us.

Jack and I decided to take career breaks for a couple of months and went travelling to Australia, New Zealand and California to escape our heartbreak and live outside our fertility nightmare for a few months. On the last day of our trip, I found out that I was pregnant but started bleeding heavily a few hours later. We managed to get back to the UK and it was confirmed that I had had another ectopic pregnancy, in my right tube this time. My body had failed again.

The doctors couldn't save my tube and it was removed a few days later. Our chances of ever conceiving naturally were gone and this was the final straw for both of us, after our seventh loss. It was now time to draw a line under this chapter and move on to the next step. We were not giving up without a fight. The end goal was a baby and if that meant giving up the dream of carrying one and being pregnant myself, then I had to accept that.

Luckily, Em told us her offer was still on the table and was excited that we had chosen to try surrogacy. She had just had her second baby, so we would need to wait until she had finished breastfeeding to go ahead but there was a lot of preparation required anyway before that could happen. We discussed everything with our doctor at our clinic and the first step was individual and group counselling. Jack and I also had to go through another round of IVF where we had two pre-genetic screening embryos frozen for when we were able to transfer to Em.

We had decided on a natural cycle so that Em only needed limited medication. A year after accepting her offer, we started the monitoring process which involved daily scans at our clinic. The first two monitoring cycles didn't go to plan for various reasons but on the third cycle in July 2019, we finally got to the day of transfer.

The next ten days were incredibly nerve-racking. I didn't know what we would do if it didn't work. The day before our test day, we all woke up with itchy feet and decided to do the test a day early. Em FaceTimed us. I was convinced it would be negative. But she held it up to reveal two lines. It had worked! Wow, we couldn't believe it. It had really worked! However, we couldn't feel any relief until an early scan could tell us that the pregnancy was growing as it should be.

A couple of weeks later, the scan showed us something that we had not seen in six years – a heartbeat. This was by far the most incredible moment we had experienced for a long time and a day none of us will ever forget. I believe the minute the sonographer said,

'There's a baby with a heartbeat' was a moment that changed me as a person and I felt a glimmer of the old me suddenly come back.

Over the next couple of months, we pretty much held our breath and had scans every few weeks to help with the anxiety. Each one showed normal growth and we had finally reached the 12-week mark. It was then that our baby started looking like a real baby. We had, at long last, got through a first trimester.

The second trimester seemed to fly by. When Em was 17 weeks pregnant, we decided to go for a private gender scan which, much to my surprise, revealed we were having a little boy. From that moment things started to feel slightly more real and I finally allowed myself to go into a baby shop and buy a few things. We felt first kicks at around 26 weeks which was magical, and soon after Jack and I started decorating the nursery.

Having had various discussions between all of us and the hospital, we decided that an elective caesarean was what felt right for our situation. In March 2020, the week before our baby was due, England was put into a national lockdown due to Covid-19. It became touch and go as to whether Jack and I were going to be allowed at the birth – it would have broken my heart had we not been. We all went into self-isolation for a week prior to give ourselves the best possible shot of being allowed at his birth.

The morning of the C-section we picked Em up. As we arrived at the hospital, all of our temperatures were checked and were normal, thank goodness. The hospital was incredibly accommodating and we were put in a private room. The morning passed and we were taken to surgery. I remember holding Em's hand from the very start of the procedure, not quite believing what was about to happen. The next thing we knew, the doctors were saying that our baby was almost here and that's when all our tears started. We played a special song that we had chosen for him and the minute our little boy was born was the most magical and surreal moment of our lives. I was worried that I would feel like he wasn't ours but those feelings never materialised. I looked at him and felt like the luckiest human in the world. I then looked at Em and felt overwhelmed with pride and amazement. He was really here and, after six years of holding my breath, I felt the weight finally lift. Our little Leo.

Our losses and fertility journey changed both Jack and I as people, in positive and negative ways. Luckily, it also made us fairly resilient and I feel blessed that I had a supportive husband, family and special friends by my side the whole time. Every person has a different story and a different level of grief, which I came to learn after spending years feeling guilty that other people were in worse situations and experiencing much later losses than we were. I may never have got to name our babies but they were still very much a part of us. Losing a pregnancy or struggling to have a baby can feel like the loneliest experience in the world, so I decided early on in our journey that being open and talking about our past, present and future was an absolute must – to help myself and hopefully others too one day. I would always advise people to talk to whomever you feel comfortable opening up to.

There will always be a small part of me that feels sad that my body couldn't carry our baby and that I will likely never experience pregnancy, giving birth, feeling my baby kick inside me or breastfeeding. However, I have now come to learn and accept they are not the sole things that make you a mother. I wake up every day and look at our blue-eyed, blonde-haired little boy and still can't believe my luck that I finally got to be a mummy. He is our miracle and fills me with joy every time he smiles. I am forever grateful that our story had a happy ending. We will also always be thankful that our amazing friend helped us – sometimes it really can take a team of people to create miracles.

I would say to any woman or man currently in the depths of their own fertility journey: do not give up on hope. Even when you have none left yourself, focus on those around you who do hold on to it for you. Miracles happen even when you have given up believing.

To Leo James – it was always you.

Born From My Heart
by Rachel Lyons

I remember the day we were told we would need IVF. We sat opposite the fertility consultant as she told us that we had unexplained infertility and we would require IVF. I had honestly thought there would be other options we could try before going down that route. I remember feeling offended that she said we were suffering 'infertility'. I was ovulating; my husband's sperm results were fine, so why were we 'infertile'? That word cut deep. With that word came so many feelings that I was not prepared for. I just needed to have some control over the situation but this is one time in life that all control is stripped from you.

The consultant told us that this was an exciting journey and to enjoy it but all I felt was fear. I was so desperate for everything to go OK and for us to have the child we longed for that the thought of it not working terrified me.

Our first round of IVF gave us three good quality embryos. We decided to have two embryos transferred and have one frozen. I was immediately attached to them; they were the closest I had ever felt to feeling pregnant. We then had to go through the agonising two-week wait to find out if I was. It was the culmination of what felt like a mammoth journey – constant hurdles, examinations, tests, injections, hormone therapy, scans and eagerly awaited phone calls from the specialist nurses. Our embryos gave us hope, they gave us a vision of what might be. I spoke to them every day of that two week period. I hoped with every part of my being that they would hold on in there and stay with me. We had been through so much to make them and we already felt like a perfect team.

At the end of the very long two-week wait, I felt like I was getting all the symptoms of pregnancy but I knew this could be due to the hormones I was taking. I remember the day that our journey came to an end: I went to the toilet and I had started to bleed. My husband was at work so I was home alone with just my dog. I just sat there in silence for quite some time, trying to muster up the courage to call him and share the sad news. That was probably one of the saddest moments. We had agreed that if anything happened, I would just call him and ask him to come home, so he knew the news was not good. I sat in my bathroom holding on to my wonderful, loving dog and sobbed like I have never done before. My world was caving in around me. Nothing could have prepared me for the sense of loss I felt following IVF. I did all the self-preservation I possibly could but when the day came that we found out it had not worked my world fell apart.

Time passed and the grieving process was all-consuming at times. Friends around me were having babies, some even having their second. I felt like I was outside, looking through the window of a club I wasn't a part of and everyone on the other side had all of the happiness that I dreamed of having.

Eventually, over a year later, we tried a second round of IVF. Sadly, once again, we went for our pregnancy blood test and it was negative. I knew in my heart that was the last go, the last chance, as I physically and emotionally couldn't endure it all again.

Grieving after IVF is so hard to explain. There is nothing tangible. It's a loss of opportunity, the loss of hopes and dreams and a future you thought was so nearly within your reach. I also felt like I had failed, as a woman, a wife, a daughter. I couldn't understand why I just couldn't hold on to those precious embryos.

It took a long time to process my grief. I slipped into a depression and I needed to speak to someone. I went to see my GP and broke down completely. I was referred for counselling, which I literally had to drag myself to, but, eventually, with time, it felt like I was closing a door but a new one was opening. A new sense of hope started to shine through. One day, my counsellor asked me if I felt I could mother any child, regardless of whether I had given birth to them. In an instant I said yes. Being a mother had become way more to me than a nine-month pregnancy and genetics. I needed to be a mother; it was embedded in my make-up.

In May 2018, my husband and I went along to an adoption open evening. I was so nervous but also so excited. After learning a great deal about the adoption process and listening to a couple who had adopted their son, we both felt like this was a path we were meant to take. It felt like the most natural thing in the world. Within a month we were assigned a social worker and so our adoption journey began.

On 6th March 2019, it was our panel day. A process where a panel of individuals, all of whom have a link to adoption on a personal or professional level, would interview us. I was so incredibly nervous. I'm usually confident at public speaking, those who know me well know I can chat a lot, but I was just so worried I wouldn't be able to get across to them how much adoption meant to me. My husband and I entered the panel room where eight people were sitting around a large table, all smiling at us. We nervously answered their questions and spoke about the journey that had led us to that moment. Eventually the nerves faded away and we were able to talk with ease about why we were ready to be parents and about the love we had to give – the life, the hope that we longed for as a family.

It was a unanimous decision from the panel – we were approved as adopters. I still remember that day with so much pride and love in my heart.

Two months passed and then the eagerly awaited phone call came; one I will never, ever forget. Our social worker told us we had been matched. My heart flipped. Our social worker asked if we could be ready quickly and without any hesitation we said yes! We had half a day's notice to prepare and get the bare essentials ready for her arrival but friends and family rallied around us, delivering their spare items to help us. We quickly realised what an amazing, kind support network we had around us.

Then the day was upon us; we both paced the house, having spent hours cleaning and rearranging the bedroom, setting up a crib next to my side of the bed, ironing freshly washed baby grows and cute baby girl outfits. It hadn't really hit me what was actually happening, I just went into immediate organisation mode. The call came from our social worker: 'We're in the car and we're on our way.' That wait felt like the longest one by far. It felt longer than the six years of longing we had endured, waiting for this very moment.

I watched out of the lounge window, feeling absolutely ready to hold our baby girl. Then I saw our social worker walking up the road with her in her arms. All I kept saying was, 'She's so tiny.' I opened the front door and I instantly felt a love that there are simply no words to describe. I felt like her face was one I had always known. Our social worker handed her over to me and said to her, 'Here is your mummy and daddy.' In an instant, our whole purpose in life changed. This little baby girl was giving us a life we had longed for, she was giving us everything, and even more, than we could have ever imagined. She was always meant for us and, just like that, it all made sense. We had been waiting all that time to be chosen for her and her for us. She may not have our biological make-up but she was born from our hearts.

I can honestly say that everything we went through was leading us to our beautiful girl. I know that in my heart for sure. My journey to motherhood may not have been the most conventional. However, I feel no different to other mothers and I feel so proud that I am an adoptive mother. The grief, the heartache – I would go through it all again in a heartbeat if I knew I was being led to her. There isn't a day that goes past where I don't thank the universe for everything that's happened to us. If I can offer hope to anyone out there going through a similar experience of loss or grief, I promise you it will be OK.

There was a time I honestly felt like my life was not worth living. I couldn't face social situations and I dreaded seeing friends as they all had their babies. That is a time I will never forget and the loss we endured will always be a part of me. However, if I could speak to myself back then, I would whisper, 'You are not a failure, you are stronger than you realise and good things are not far away.'

First Comes Love, Then Comes Marriage, Then Comes a Miscarriage
by Vanessa Haye

My journey to motherhood to date has been far from a fairy tale.

If Disney ever needed another story with a 'spin' then mine would certainly match the criteria. Except that you may have noticed that mothers as fully fledged characters are rarely present in the landscape of Disney fairy tales. The portrayal of family adventure and misfortunes also very typically transitions into 'happy ever after' endings as opposed to mirroring my own personal experiences of infertility and a rather non-whimsical journey to motherhood.

My husband and I spent three and a half years trying for a baby, as well as losing the babies that we hoped would be a part of the family I dreamed of. This is a journey that many other women have been on but one we rarely, if ever, see depicted. A lack of representation at the time when I needed to 'see me' most made me feel invisible and excluded from the motherhood narrative. But, despite that, even in being and feeling unseen, I still believed in a joyful ending – with or even without children.

I was raised one of four daughters in a suburban area of north London by first-generation working-class Ghanaian immigrants – memories of my childhood are full of moments that I will cherish forever and undoubtedly shaped my desire to be a mother one day. Throughout my childhood and into my independent late-teenage years, my parents worked night and day to provide for our family and give us the best life. Even though I would say they didn't acquire much of what they deserved, they would do anything to give my sisters and I what we needed.

I have particularly vivid memories of our family Christmases. Each year, our little tree was adorned with a colourful array of biblical figurines from the nativity scene and iridescent rainbow lights. My most favourite ornament was a gold-papered polystyrene cube with a bow, imitating a mini gift. I loved it because our tree wasn't ordinarily the picturesque type paraded in catalogues and surrounded with an abundance of gifts. However, one year, my inquisitive sisters and I ventured into our parents' bedroom and to our surprise their floor was covered with shopping bags filled with Barbie dolls and Cinderella slippers. It was as if our scrapbooks plastered with our Argos wish list had come alive! Our parents had worked tirelessly and would do anything to make us feel loved and like the princesses they always affirmed us to be.

These fond memories are what led to my self-constructed idea of how I imagined my journey to becoming a mother would go. I longed for the day when I too would have children of my own to protect and, moreover, grew increasingly moved at the thought of giving my prospective children the life that I yearned for but didn't have, even when I knew my parents worked fervently to make us happy.

My parents had shown many times over what unconditional love looked like and I took a leaf out of their book at Christmas in 2015 when I made a decision to undergo fertility treatment as it seemed at the time to be the only way I would get pregnant. My fertility consultant had told me that my chances of conceiving naturally were very low due to my past history and ongoing issues of irregular and at most times absent periods. I was informed that the only likely way I would achieve a pregnancy was by assisted fertility treatments such as intrauterine insemination (IUI) or in vitro fertilisation (IVF).

By this point, I had already been through eight gruelling and unsuccessful cycles of clomiphene as well as a failed IUI cycle, so the thought of having to have multiple daily injections, experiencing medical menopause at the tender age of 27 and fluctuating weight gain did not deter me. I was prepared to go through anything at all in the hope of being awarded my very own title as a 'mother', despite the fact that IVF could not guarantee I would graduate to this seemingly higher rank of womanhood.

This unconventional route to conception was rarely discussed in my community. As a Black woman, I was supposedly 'hyper fertile', someone who could and 'should' get pregnant just by looking at my husband, and so to avoid any unwanted scepticism or advice, my husband and I accepted that we would go through treatment without telling anyone apart from our close family members. Although this was extremely isolating, throughout the treatment cycle my resilience grew and I became more and more unfazed. All that mattered was our quest to become pregnant and finally have a baby of our very own that we could take home to start the family life we dreamed of.

In November 2016, we were ecstatic and felt incredibly blessed to learn that our first IVF cycle had worked.

Owing to my obsession with having our first family Christmas, I was excited at being near to finally accomplishing my Pinterest-inspired Christmas pregnancy announcement to our close family and friends. At the point at which we planned to tell everyone our news, I would have been just shy of ten weeks pregnant. Considering all that we had endured to get to this point, we were taking a big risk by making our announcement before our first dating scan and when we were not officially 'out of the woods'. However, I was so relieved to finally take hold of the baton in this race to motherhood. I was more concerned with proving that my body could achieve a pregnancy – it was as if this baby was not only ours but the baby everyone else was waiting for.

Sadly, at six weeks we lost our baby. My husband and I were devasted to say the least and I was plagued with feelings of inadequacy and failure. I felt like a defective woman because not only was I unable to conceive naturally but even with help, my body couldn't maintain a pregnancy.

Just like any fairy tale, this was the point in our story where there was a sudden cruel twist and I felt like I'd been forced into a position of humility where I had to challenge my own pronatalist assumptions pertaining to motherhood. Feeling so close but yet so far away made me come to the understanding that becoming a mother or parents was in fact a privilege and a gift as opposed to a guaranteed destination.

The hardest part of the grieving process was having to grit our teeth at the unwarranted but well-meaning comments from our church 'family', friends and close relatives who were none the wiser as to what we had been through and would regularly ask us when we planned to start a family, as if being husband and wife doesn't already constitute that. The harder moments were when others brazenly enquired whether we were expecting a baby, when in fact my ever-changing rotund appearance was a result of being injected with fertility hormones during our second IVF cycle that we started in the spring of 2017.

This time, we were fortunately able to undergo a frozen embryo transfer cycle using embryos from our first IVF cycle; I was so relieved that I didn't have to go through the egg retrieval process again. At this point of our journey, we started to find meaning and contentment. We always looked for the silver lining as opposed to waiting to land on 'cloud nine'. Our Christian faith and belief in God kept us going through our second cycle and we agreed to continue praying and hoping for our miracle rainbow baby. We also guarded our hearts just in case we were met with further disappointments. Experiencing so much loss and heartache sometimes made it difficult for us to believe that things would work out in the end.

Fortunately, our second cycle was successful and resulted in our second pregnancy but, once again, there were difficult challenges along the way. I experienced many weeks of severe bleeding and so, even after seeing our baby's flicker of heartbeat at our six-week dating scan, we continued to pay for private scans for further reassurance and also as a way of reaffirmation, because each time we approached a new week we could hardly believe that we were getting closer to meeting our precious baby.

In February 2018, after a long, painful and hard labour, we finally had our beautiful baby boy Sebastian. As we settled into this new stage of life and parenthood, it was easy to forget the journey we had been on to get to here. We could attest to what people meant when they had encouraged us that all we had been through would be worth it in the end.

At times, this happy ending was so euphoric that I started to become concerned with how long this feeling of bliss would last once our son began to grow up. Although this wasn't something we needed to worry about just yet, we could never ignore the uncertainty of whether we would be able to continue to grow our family and were often asked if we had plans to have another baby.

Unexpectedly, in August 2019, we found out that we were expecting again after conceiving naturally but sadly we lost our miracle baby and I almost lost my life as a result of a ruptured ectopic pregnancy, which also meant the removal of my left fallopian tube. It was hard to make sense of this tragic loss because I was subjected to the double-edged sword of losing a baby as well as part of my fertility and my biology that I had always relied upon to perfect my ideal biography – a happy home full of children.

After spending months recovering from surgery, we finally got to bury our tiny baby in December 2019. In this moment of déjà vu, we spent yet another Christmas as a family grieving but we also chose to hold on to the glimmer of hope. We were grateful that my life was saved; I couldn't possibly fathom that my son was so close to being left without a mother and my husband without his wife.

As I conclude, for now we remain a family of five, because we will never forget our two angel babies. We are determined to take joy in what we now perceive to be an adventure as opposed to a journey. I say this because, in hindsight, my personal highs and lows were all very significant parts of the process to becoming a mother. Even before I was able to finally hold a living baby in my arms, I understood that having the title of a mother was not limited to my ability to carry a child but rather transcended my physical capabilities.

I once read that a mother's love is unrivalled because many other women like me who face difficulty conceiving or even maintaining a pregnancy have already demonstrated that we would do anything for the child that we are yet to meet, even when our story does not end with holding our baby in our arms.

I personally have learned that however your story begins and unfolds, everyone's journey to motherhood, or even 'otherhood', is unique and whatever happens in the end isn't always necessarily the end but perhaps a new beginning and path of hope. This certainly was the case for me.

Loved and Wanted
by Zara Dawson

On 26th October 2018, we said goodbye to our darling son Jesse. We'd made the heart-breaking decision to terminate our pregnancy after being told he was simply 'incompatible with life' due to a rare defect called body stalk anomaly. This is, I was to learn later, a 'termination for medical reasons' or 'TFMR', something that, at the time of his diagnosis, I'd never even heard of, let alone thought I'd ever have to go through. I am so thankful to Elle for inviting me to tell my story within this book, to not only raise awareness around TFMR but hopefully to offer some support and comfort to others who find themselves going through this devastating loss.

My husband Lex and I started trying for a baby in 2014. After a year with no luck, I went to my GP who referred us for IVF. Within a few months, the cycle was underway and I had started the injections. We were overjoyed when we learned it had been successful. However, the pregnancy was incredibly complicated. I developed severe OHSS (ovarian hyperstimulation syndrome) from the drugs. Fluid leaked from my ovaries into my abdomen and around my lungs, making it incredibly difficult to breathe. I was petrified and had no idea how I was meant to grow a baby when my body was struggling so much from the IVF.

I suffered five incidents of ovarian torsion, which is when the ovaries twist round on themselves causing excruciating pain, and at ten weeks pregnant I needed emergency surgery. I initially begged the consultant not to operate but after hearing him comment to the nurse 'this lady is in real trouble', I knew I didn't have a choice. They told us there was a high chance that we would miscarry during the procedure and, as I was wheeled down to the operating theatre, that's what I tried to prepare myself for. To wake up and find I had lost my longed-for baby. The scan after I came round from the operation was petrifying. I fully expected to hear the words 'I'm so sorry but there's no heartbeat'. Instead we saw our baby dancing away on the screen!

I spent almost three months in hospital during the pregnancy. Those were incredibly lonely days, full of fear and anxiety. I didn't buy anything for the baby. I truly never thought we'd get to take him home and I thought it would be easier after we'd lost him if there weren't constant reminders everywhere.

Jax was born at 36 weeks. The birth was extremely traumatic, ending up with me in surgery for hours and Jax being taken into the NICU. I'll never forget being wheeled to my bed on the postnatal ward. All the other mothers in the room had their babies lying beside them in a cot. The cot beside my bed was empty. I feel bereft, traumatised, frightened yet nobody asked how I was.

I spent every minute I could with Jax, just sitting beside his cot on the NICU unit, holding his little hand, trying to bond with him and get him stronger so he could come out and be with me. I so needed him. I'd been in hospital for almost five weeks this time and I was really struggling with living in a tiny bay, dealing with my postnatal hormones and missing my baby. I had barely any milk yet would force myself to sit up all hours of the night trying to express. Looking back, I think I was punishing myself – I felt I'd done such an awful job carrying him throughout the pregnancy that I HAD to provide him with milk. Surely that was the least I could do?

Thankfully, a few stressful weeks later, he was well enough to come out. We left the hospital and began our life as a family of three. I was still in shock our boy was here. After being told on a few separate occasions during the pregnancy it looked like we were losing him, he had proven them all wrong. We had made it.

After about a year of motherhood, I started counselling with the incredible Flora Saxby at Petals, a charity that provides specialist support to those who have suffered baby loss, to try to process all I'd been through as I just couldn't seem to move forward. I was getting flashbacks and my anxiety was in overdrive. We knew we wanted to try for a sibling for Jax and, after a year of working with her, I felt I was ready to try again.

We started our first frozen cycle in 2018. It was an absolute walk in the park compared to the fresh IVF cycle we had done three years previously! I simply used an ovulation stick at home daily until I got a positive result, then headed into the clinic six days later to have a transfer! And that was it. Lex went into the cycle with a lot of trepidation but I had the mindset that nothing could be as bad as what I went through the first time. How wrong I was.

To our absolute amazement, the cycle worked. From very early on, I was floored with severe nausea – but I absolutely loved it! I felt like my body was trying to let me know that everything was OK and the baby was growing well. I was scanned regularly because of my previous issues when I was pregnant with Jax and we loved seeing our little one growing week by week. Jax loved nothing more than rubbing my bump and telling me he was going to be a big brother!

Then came the news that changed everything. I'll never forget 'that' scan. We were watching the screen as our baby was kicking and waving away. The sonographer told us everything looked good and asked me to sit in the waiting room so I could speak with the nurse about getting some anti-sickness medication.

At 12:07, I text my mum and sister: 'Scan fine. Baby is VERY active!' At 12:25, however, I sent another message: 'They just told me they've found a pouch of fluid on his stomach which means his stomach hasn't closed. Devastated.'

Within those 18 minutes, my world completely collapsed. I was alone when the sonographer called me back into the room. I remember watching her mouth moving and not being able to take in what she was saying. She told me there was something wrong but to come back in two weeks for another scan. I left the room in a complete daze and asked to speak to a consultant.

I waited at the early pregnancy unit for six hours until a consultant could see me. Six hours of constant Googling. Six hours of sitting on my own in a room, sobbing. I felt sick with worry. Looking back now, I think deep down, I knew. I kept seeing the words 'termination' come up on the pages I was Googling and I just couldn't get my head round it. I couldn't 'terminate' my pregnancy. My baby was alive and kicking.

Up until that point, I'd thought baby loss meant miscarriage and stillbirth. I'd never even considered there could be another way in which you could lose your baby. When I finally managed to speak with the consultant, she told me it could be one of three things. The pouch of fluid they'd found on the scan was indicating that some of Jesse's organs were outside of his body. Depending on which organs these were, it was possible that this could be treated with operations soon after birth. However, if it was something called body stalk anomaly, this was untreatable and the baby would be deemed 'incompatible with life'. But, she said, 'This is so rare, we aren't dealing with this one.'

I travelled back home in a total daze. I remember looking at people who were heading on a night out and wanted to scream at them. They looked so happy and carefree and my world was crumbling. The next day, I booked a private scan at the Portland Hospital in London. After being scanned for quite some time, the sonographer put down the scanner and said, 'I'm so, so sorry.' They told me Jesse did in fact have body stalk anomaly. Even if he did survive the pregnancy, he would die during birth or shortly afterwards. His foot had also started to protrude out of the amniotic sac, putting my health at risk. I remained eerily silent while Lex sobbed beside me.

Back home, I broke down, sobbing harder than I ever have before. I stayed up until 3:30am, continuing

my research. When I read there were no recorded sur-
vivors of body stalk anomaly, I knew what we were
facing. I cried myself to sleep that night, praying that
Jesse would die naturally to alleviate some of the shattering guilt I'd started to feel.

Over the next couple of days, we had a number of
scans with consultants from the Foetal Medicine Unit
at the hospital to make sure the diagnosis was correct
and to help us decide our next steps. After the final
detailed scan, they confirmed the previous findings
from the Portland Hospital – that Jesse was so unwell,
he would not survive. His left leg was bent up behind
his back, he had tumours at the base of his spine and
every organ was outside of his body – apart from his
heart which had dropped down to his abdomen as
there were no other organs to hold it in place. Despite
this, it was beating perfectly until the very end.

They allowed us an hour-long scan where we
recorded the heartbeat and filmed his tiny, perfect face.
He had the same button nose as Jax. He really was so,
so beautiful. I didn't ever want that scan to end. That
was the last time I would see my baby. My boy Jesse.
But we could also see the extent of his anomaly and
knew we were making the only decision we felt we
could. I whispered the words, 'OK, you can stop now,'

to the consultant. And that was that. The last time we'd ever see our baby boy's perfect little face.

I was told I could have a medical termination the following week. This is where you are admitted into the hospital, given medication to induce labour and give birth. I was present years earlier when my nephew was born sleeping and I just couldn't bear to be back in a room where that happened again. I was also warned that the sight of Jesse would not be one I would want to remember. I decided to opt for a surgical termination. The hospital wouldn't be able to facilitate this for me so I was sent away with a leaflet for ARC – the Antenatal Results and Choices charity, which advises and supports parents in situations such as ours – and one for Marie Stopes abortion clinic. And that's it. I was left to call around and book in my termination myself. I immediately called ARC and spoke to an amazing lady called Jane. The second she answered, I just cried down the phone at her, rambling away, but she calmed me down and talked me through my choices. I'd never heard of ARC before but, then again, I'd never been faced with terminating my much-wanted pregnancy before.

The following day, I set about calling round the Marie Stopes clinics to see where I could get booked in. They found a space for me in a week's time at a clinic in south London. I was concerned as this procedure wasn't being performed in a hospital and all of my previous gynaecological surgeries had had one complication or another. I asked what would happen if something unexpected was to happen during the surgery. The lady replied, 'We'll call an ambulance and blue light you to the nearest hospital.' That didn't sit particularly well with me. Next, I asked how I could get my baby's body back to my hospital as we were having genetic testing performed. She told me cheerily, 'We'll give it to you on the day. But don't worry, it won't be in a see-through box.' I put the phone down and felt so uneasy, yet it didn't seem I had a choice. But then the clinic called me back and said because of my gynaecological history, they weren't sure they would perform the surgery for me after all. Where did this leave me?

I fought with the hospital for two weeks and finally they agreed they would perform the surgery there instead. For a brief moment it felt like a victory. Then came the realisation that I now knew the date that Jesse would die. Those two weeks, when I knew what was coming to my baby, were unbearable. I'd bump into friends who would congratulate me on the pregnancy.

I'd say thank you, then walk away and break down. If only they knew.

The day of the termination was one I will never forget. Just beyond heart-breaking and full of guilt. I sobbed as I was put to sleep and I saw that the anaesthetist was crying too. I kept telling the surgical team that I really didn't want to be doing this but the baby was so poorly. I just wanted them to know that my baby was SO loved and wanted. The whole procedure was over fairly quickly and I was back home that afternoon.

In the weeks and months that followed, I learned that TFMR is the baby loss that no one speaks of. It is far more common that you'd expect, with over 5,000 babies lost to TFMR every single year. Yet, until now, there has been so little support out there for those parents who have gone through it. In my darkest days, I made a pact to myself that, as soon as I felt strong enough, I would speak about what I'd been through to try to improve this and get rid of the stigma that is so often attached to it. We deserve support as much as any mother who has been through a loss. After all, we lost our babies too.

Chapter 15

A Christmas Miracle?

I SAT BLINKING AS I STARED AT WHAT SEEMED LIKE AN IMPOSSIBLE RESULT IN THE TINY WINDOW ON THE STICK THAT LAY IN MY HANDS. It was 6:30am on a crisp, early December morning and I had run to the bathroom to pee on a stick for the first time in what had felt like an eternity. I had been waiting for my period to arrive so that I could call the clinic and we could get started once more. It hadn't showed up. So I waited a couple of days, and then a couple more, but now I was done with waiting and I just wanted to get the inevitable disappointment over with so that I could call them to say it was late again and I didn't know why.

We were due to go into London that day for my husband's birthday celebrations, for a special lunch we had booked in an attempt to cheer ourselves up after all of the trials and tribulations of 2019. Our little shot at being festive. I didn't want this uncertainty, this strange feeling I had to cloud the day, so I rummaged in the back of the bathroom cupboard and quickly grabbed a test I had bought in advance of our freeze-all round. I didn't tell Nico what I was doing, I waited until he was downstairs making morning tea and stealthily crept into the bathroom so that the deed would be done and we could get on with our day.

Except now time seemed to stop still. In the palm of my hand were two lines. Pregnant. But *how?* (I should probably point out at this point that obviously I do know *how*, you don't get this far into a fertility journey and not understand the basics of how a baby is traditionally made. What I didn't understand was how *now?* WHY NOW?!) My head was spinning, my heart was in my mouth and nothing seemed to make sense. I ran downstairs and into the kitchen, to the surprise of my husband who looked almost as shocked as I felt.

'What's wrong?' he said.

I didn't speak. Instead I thrust the test into his hands and watched for a few moments as his eyes tried to focus on what they were looking at, and his brain tried to compute what it all meant.

'I don't understand . . . ?' he began, looking at me with an expression that was more than puzzled.

'Neither do I,' I replied. 'Surprise!'

Needless to say, we both hugged and sobbed. I won't ever forget that moment. It was as if the universe, after everything, had just chosen to say, 'There you go. Have this . . .'

It felt like an impossible dream, achieved at a moment when we hadn't even been looking for it. We had been so, *so* focused on getting to the next step, the next hurdle to cross. We got ready to go out and I kept checking and double-checking the test result as it lay resting on my dressing table, smiling each time when the result still clearly read the same. Pregnant.

It felt as though we went about the rest of our day in a bubble of complete bliss. I found myself swinging from utter elation, daring to imagine this could be our time, back to that crippling fear that always seemed to take over in the next breath. We spent our day in London as we had planned to: we had lunch, looked around the shops as things were starting to get a bit festive – and generally grinned like Cheshire cats. I sat and smiled across the table at Nico as he enjoyed a birthday beer and I sipped my sparkling water. The festive lights in Bond Street twinkled and every busker on every corner seemed to be playing romantic Christmas classics.

Hang on a minute . . . could it be? Did I actually, for the first time in years, feel a genuine spark of happiness in the lead up to Christmas?! I didn't care if it was short-lived even, I wanted to grasp this feeling and bottle it. I had finally found my festive cheer again! As we walked back over the footbridge to Waterloo and gazed across the water at how beautiful London appeared that day, we took a *very* cheesy photo because we wanted to hold on to that moment of happiness forever, just in case.

It really did feel like a Christmas miracle. It didn't feel real. I tested each day after it and every test still stared back at me with a glaring positive. We decided to keep it to ourselves for the next week or so as I couldn't bear to tempt fate (impossible, I know). I did, of course, call the clinic to tell them. After all, they had been expecting my call to start treatment. I got through to the nurses on my first attempt (that *never* happened!) and, by some strange twist of fate, it was that same kind nurse who picked up, who had gone through her own long fertility journey. It was as if it was meant to be. I told her our news and I immediately heard her voice crack. She was crying. I was crying too. I could tell she was so happy for us, that she knew exactly what it felt like to be in that position after everything, because she had been there too. She asked me to keep them updated and told me she would inform the consultant that we wouldn't be needing to proceed with the planned treatment round.

The phone call felt like a dream. I had always heard and read stories from other people who had endured rounds of drugs and IVF with no success and then, one day, just fell pregnant. It had always felt like reading magical fairy tales of happily-ever-afters that couldn't possibly be true. As if these kinds of things only existed in myth and legend within the fertility community and surely no one, *ever*, just ended up pregnant without treatment? Yet, here I was, pregnant, and not a needle in sight.

When we told our parents, the shock and confusion on their faces was also pretty easy to read.

I said to my mum and dad on FaceTime: 'So, we've decided not to go ahead with our round of IVF.' I watched as my mum's puzzled face looked crestfallen. 'Because we don't need to . . . because I'm pregnant.'

Both of their faces changed instantly, to wide smiles and then tears. I won't *ever* forget it. It felt like the best early Christmas present we could have given them. Telling our siblings over Christmas felt like a dream, too. I always imagined we would be able to tell everyone (the news I knew they had all longed for too, after losing Teddy) at such a special time of year. It made it feel even more like a fairy tale.

Of course, I didn't believe in fairy tales or happily ever after anymore, not really. Not after everything it had taken to get us to this point. The reality of it all hit when the Early Pregnancy Unit called me after I had called my consultant's secretary to let her know our news. She said they would arrange an early scan for me. When they called a day or two later, the reality set in. I actually didn't want an early scan. It had caused too much confusion, waiting and heartache in our last experience of loss. I wasn't ready for that again. So, we declined having it before Christmas because I wanted to be able to get to a point where any pregnancy and, most importantly, a heartbeat, would be definitively seen or not. I didn't want that familiar weight of confusion or doubt hanging over us at 'the most wonderful time of the year'. As someone who has had enough cancelled Christmases, I didn't need another. We were just starting to get that long-lost Christmas spirit back after all. We decided to keep it for ourselves, to host and enjoy, and hope for the best while we waited for January and another new year to be upon us.

Chapter 16

I Can See a Rainbow

WE WERE IN CORNWALL WITH FAMILY OVER NEW YEAR
WHEN SICKNESS BEGAN TO TRULY KICK IN. By my es-
timation, I wasn't even eight weeks yet but the nausea was *real*. I remember my sister-in-law saying to
me as I lay on the bench seat in the kitchen, 'But this
is good news, isn't it? A good sign, surely?' As I lay
there in my fog of sickness, I bloody well hoped she
was right. Surely these signs and symptoms *had* to be
laced with the promise of good news? I thought back
to my last two pregnancies, after Teddy. During the
first, I has felt so unwell from about week seven and
yet that baby had been too poorly to live. The second,
after IVF, had literally seen me clinging to the bed with

253

sickness, wishing the world would stop spinning. Yet those babies had already had their fate decided too. What would make this any different?

The only thing that seemed to ease the cloud of nausea was fresh air (well, that and more beige food) and so we walked and we walked. The blustery sea air and long beach walks brought me back to life. Feeling the spray on my face and like I could actually breathe in – properly, fully, for the first time in months – felt wonderful. Would we actually be facing a happy year ahead, 12 months of happy events and perhaps not even an IVF needle in sight? I tried my hardest to enjoy each moment. I savoured each day that I woke up and was still pregnant.

Though I still found myself filled with dread at each trip to the bathroom. Would there be blood? Would it be the moment that marked the beginning of the end, again? It was as though I had jumped straight from the endless cycle of *wanting* to get pregnant again to now knowing I was and fearing every day that it would be over. Once again, when it's going on inside you, you simply cannot ignore it. You can't just 'think of something else' or 'try not to worry'. It's there, a constant, never further than your next thought.

When I was first expecting Teddy, I can remember being filled with pure joy in those first weeks of knowing. Yes, there was sickness, but my excitement seemed to overshadow any other emotion. I had no fears, no doubt in my mind over whether that baby inside me would live or die, I just enjoyed it. This time was unrecognisably different; every day was already beginning to feel like the slowest I had ever lived through. I had once heard someone describing their experience of pregnancy after loss as running a marathon, through treacle, and they were pretty bloody accurate.

As we made our way back home from Cornwall, it dawned on me that our first scan would be in just a few short days. I had been so set on just making it through Christmas and New Year I hadn't allowed myself to think ahead to what might happen next, in that scan room. The 'scanxiety' began to set in. It being January again, it was easy to hide – no one expected to see me and Nico was back to work.

The night before the scan I didn't sleep, running through every outcome in my head over and over, all of them worse than the one before. As we walked into the hospital and to the EPU that morning, I was pretty sure I was set to vomit, and it wasn't from pregnancy sickness. I was shaking like a leaf and, as we sat waiting, neither of us said a word, we were both crippled with fear. Not how most couples envisage their first scan of a longed-for baby, I'm sure.

We were accompanied into the room by the kind EPU nurse who had seen so much of me the previous year. The same one who had sat with me during my full and final 'I've lost the plot moment' after I was told that my miscarriage might have been not only molar but cancer. She knew what this moment meant to us; I could see it on her face. She kept reassuring me and said, 'I won't leave you, I'll be right here.'

The same consultant sonographer who had first diagnosed my missed miscarriage held the scanner in her hand as I asked for the screens we could see to be off and turned away. The room was dimly lit and deathly quiet; tears were already streaming down my face as I clenched hold of my husband's hand with a vice-like grip, clinging on for dear life, on the precipice of falling back into that deep, dark hole. My jeans already didn't fit me, there *had* to be a growing baby in there, but I couldn't bring myself to believe it.

As the silence broke, I won't forget the words the doctor said when she scanned over my tummy that first time (no dildo wand required, I'm afraid), as if to reassure me the very first second that she got the chance: 'The baby is fine.'

Tears streamed down both of our faces, and the face of the nurse who had comforted us so many times before, as the sound of a little heartbeat pumped so loudly through that monitor, filling the room with that joyous sound. A sound that we had hoped for, for so long.

The nurse looked at me, beaming and crying, and said, 'See, she promised you healthy babies before retirement, didn't she?'

She had remembered that day, and that conversation too, the one that had kept me clinging to hope when I felt like hope was all but gone. My tears turned to laughter and a smile so wide I felt my face might crack. 'Thank you. Thank you so much,' was all I could hear myself repeating over and over to everyone in that room.

I felt as though we were both (actually, all *three* of us) walking on air as we stepped out of the hospital that day. Even though the worry was still there, we had seen a baby, heart beating, and nothing could top that as a start to our year.

A day or two later, I picked up the phone to 'NO CALLER ID' and I knew it would be the hospital. My usual consultant was at the end when I answered and it felt so good to hear her reassuring voice.

'I know you've been for a scan already but I just wanted to call you ahead of your next one with me in a couple of weeks to say I was thrilled to hear your news. I got the letter in my tray just before Christmas and honestly it was the best present I could have hoped for.'

Her words reduced me to tears (again). I kept saying thank you. I couldn't believe she had felt the need to call me personally to say that. She really was in our corner, fighting this with us, and I felt she wanted it almost as much as we did. The discussion quickly turned to *What next?* and it was agreed that at our next scan we would also have a harmony blood test, to test for any chromosomal abnormalities. I quickly learned that there was going to be no stone left unturned in this pregnancy. Everything felt as though it would be checked and double-checked. I supposed not only because of Teddy and my obstetric history, to check the welfare of the baby, but equally for our peace of mind. The anxiety about the next steps and tests was already mounting and I was becoming familiar with the ebb and flow of the worry in between appointments and phone calls as they came and went.

Before that next scan, I had to get through my first appointment with a midwife. It was something I had dreaded. Last time we hadn't made it that far, the time before I had made two appointments and with Teddy we had made it right the way through and ended it with midwives visiting the house as I sat there on the end of my bed, crying. I didn't think I could physically manage to walk into the doctor's surgery and sit in that room again; everything about it felt so triggering. It began to feel as though doing any of those things in a familiar setting, with even a hint of connection to my previous experiences, would somehow 'tempt fate' with this baby. Of course, I knew that wasn't true, and was entirely impossible, but the mind is *such* a powerful thing and it begins to convince you that things might go wrong again if they are repeated in the same sequence. I felt the urge to make everything different this time, unrecognisable almost. *Different baby, different experience, different outcome* is what I tried to repeat to myself. It felt as though it would be the only way I could make it through each milestone without completely losing my shit, and we were still only in the first trimester . . .

When I called the midwife's office to make my first appointment, I explained that I needed to see someone who I would be able to see every time. I knew that wasn't always possible, and it hadn't happened in my pregnancy with Teddy, but the thought of having to go over and over my history with each visit was just too much to contemplate. I needed someone who knew it all, from the start, and could be there to hold my hand throughout. I was referred to a community midwife team in the next village, meaning all of my appointments would be with (hopefully) one midwife and that she would also be at the birth. Later that week, a midwife called me and I was able to tell her everything on the phone, start to finish, before I had to sit in front of her, blubbing with the whole sorry tale.

It felt easier this way, somehow, as when I saw them they would know everything and there would be no reason for me to make excuses for myself or explain why I wasn't grinning from ear to ear with excitement at each appointment. I just needed them to understand that it would be hard and that most of the time I couldn't answer the question 'How are you feeling?' because, for the most part, the answer was too complex and certainly too difficult to articulate.

I had spent so long wishing I was pregnant again, longing for that positive test, that first scan, that heartbeat. I hadn't ever given a thought to what it might be like to finally get there, what it might feel like to make it through each day, another week, another appointment. I hadn't contemplated the crippling anxiety, the fear that lived inside me with each day passing, or how triggering I could find the simplest things. It was as if I was constantly waiting for the next thing to spring up and surprise me with a new wave of emotion. I began to feel guilty for this baby, that this pregnancy would never be filled with that pure, unadulterated happiness and ignorant bliss that I had experienced first time around. I was grieving a pregnancy experience that saw me pondering thoughts that were nothing more than 'Boy or girl?' or 'What should we buy?' Instead, I began to be tortured by 'Will my baby die, again?'

The midwife was kind and understanding. She let me answer all of the questions in my own time and recognised that even stepping through that process of answering questions and ticking boxes might be an extremely hard one. At the end of my first appointment, I came away feeling like this would be a completely different experience and that they were putting all of the puzzle pieces into place to ensure that it would be. It was a weight off my mind, one less thing in the plethora of things that I had to worry about.

At our next scan we went through similar emotions as the first. A silent wait, screens turned away, no words spoken until a baby with a beating heart was seen. I was beginning to understand that this was how it was set to be this time. Just wanting everything to be OK. The baby had a slight hernia at this point, something that the consultant told us was perfectly normal and would correct itself by the next scan, something we didn't need to worry about. So, naturally, I worried myself sick and Googled myself senseless in the two weeks between scans.

Every scan report they handed me I studied in detail, every measurement I scrutinised and compared. I felt the need to try to understand everything and what it might mean in case I spotted something that might be considered a risk. Gone were the days where I just took the scan picture and stared at it lovingly. Ultimately, it was an exhausting way to exist and I knew I couldn't go on looking for things that *might* be wrong. I tried my best to put those worries to bed but it was proving to be an impossible task.

I knew that no amount of talking therapy would ever correct those thoughts or take them away. The image of my lifeless son being whisked away from my bedside that night, four years ago, in the maternity ward, was one that I could play over and over so vividly and will haunt me forever. The thought of even stepping foot in that ward again terrified me. It wasn't something I was able to think ahead to at this point; getting to that stage felt a million miles away.

After the scan, I also had my harmony blood test and we were set to have the normal combined screening too (which is there to detect Down Syndrome, but also other chromosomal differences that might mean a baby could not survive) but this one would give an earlier and more accurate result. I hoped it might take some more worry out of the equation. The blood test was quick and simple, no more invasive than a usual test – it was the wait that was agonising: almost two weeks of not knowing. In that time, I convinced myself it would be bad news (this was becoming a recurring theme, you'll notice) and I worked out ways in which we would break the news to our parents. This was, thankfully, more wasted energy on what-ifs, as the call came in from the hospital screening office to confirm that everything had come back normal and there was no risk of any of the known chromosomal disorders. I thanked the nurse who called me, over and over. She sounded a little perplexed by my enthusiasm but she had no idea how much getting over that hurdle had meant to us.

The next scan was now just days away as the wait for results from the last one had taken a while. It was as if the bubble of celebration was burst by the instant onset of scanxiety again. When would it end? Never, I knew that was the answer. The next scan only ever seemed to be more worrying than the last. I was almost 13 weeks along so I knew this would be the one where they began actively looking for things that might be wrong, where the measurements and position of things began telling vital information. I watched silently as the scan began, taking in every detail and asking questions as she went. I thought back to our first scan with Teddy when I had been just over 12 weeks, how we had laughed and smiled and left on cloud nine. It all felt so familiar, but worlds apart. Of course, we were so happy to see this little one still wriggling around on the screen, full of life, but we were also scared this time. It was as if happiness and heartbreak ran alongside one another, hand in hand. We wanted to believe in the best, because we could see the best thing that had happened to us in a long time right there in front of our eyes. But the fear of losing something so precious was unbearable. I think that unless you have experienced the loss of a baby, first hand, it is almost impossible to explain to someone just what kind of emotions rush over you when you have to go through things like detailed scans. Time just seems to stand still as you wait for the verdict.

Once again, everything was fine. She kept reassuring me, 'Baby looks healthy and normal. I'm happy.' I tried to keep playing those words over and over in my head, *healthy and normal*, as if she was happy, I should be too. We had four weeks to make to our next scan – how on earth was I going to make it another four weeks? Two had proved torturous enough. Scans were strange to experience, as we left on a temporary high, in a bubble of happiness, sure that we would bring a baby home at the end of this. Then slowly, over the days that followed, that happiness was chipped away by doubt, by questions and by fear, until over a two-week period it dwindled away to almost nothing and I needed it to be topped up by another image of the baby still doing well in there. I began to wish more than ever that I had been designed as a Teletubby so I could just switch on the screen when I wanted and check in on this little one to see that everything was still OK.

In February, it was still relatively easy to hide from everyone. I had never been so thankful that I worked from home, or that there seemed to be so many winter colds flying around that I could easily make up an illness at the drop of a hat (when really I just felt nauseous. Yes, still). I got to about 14 weeks by the time I tentatively began to tell a few friends our happy news. I braced myself each time, as I was never sure how to handle congratulations. It wasn't that I wasn't happy, or thrilled in fact, but I just felt that I could wait for congratulations to come when we brought this baby home. I knew people meant well, that they were excited for us, beyond excited it seemed in many cases! Most friends began with, 'I didn't even know you were starting treatment again?' At which point I would explain the story of the miracle baby that landed in our lives early December, usually met with more squeals of delight and disbelief.

Everyone, of course, loves a happy ending, but to me this seemed so far away from that just yet. There's never a happy ending after you lose a child; the arrival of another, or even *ten* more children, does not simply erase the one that came before. I didn't like that turn of phrase. I could see happiness, a different kind of happiness, on the horizon, within touching distance. But it wouldn't be an ending, just the beginning of a new chapter.

Chapter 17

Everything Changes But You

AS WINTER STARTED TO COME TO AN END, HIDING AWAY BECAME LESS EASY THAN IT HAD BEEN, AS PEOPLE STARTED TO ASK ME IF I WANTED TO MEET UP FOR COFFEE/WALKS/SHOPPING (INSERT ANY RANDOM ACTIVITY HERE). Granted, it had been our decision to only tell a few select people for fear of what might lie ahead but, as a result, I felt a bit like a (big) walking secret.

I had also used the first weeks of the year to get organised and plan a few little things to look forward to; it was my way of trying to break up the milestones, the scans and the general anxiety that was crashing from week to week. The first was a break in Norfolk with my parents towards the end of February, a few days to escape from it all and to hide a little longer. After that, we had booked a few days in Venice for our wedding anniversary and my birthday in April. In May we would be off to France for our friend's wedding. It felt wonderful to have some lovely trips mapped out in front of us, even just to break up the worry.

We enjoyed fish and chips and blustery beach walks in north Norfolk; it was just the tonic at that time of year. My almost four-month bump was beginning to pop and I was once more welcomed into the world of dungarees and stretch waistbands to ensure comfort. My hunger was, quite frankly, next level. I remembered it had been with Teddy too; needing a constant bank of snack foods on hand at all times to keep the nausea at bay. I also developed an outrageously sweet tooth around this time and remember feeling absolutely delighted when we stumbled across an old-fashioned sweet shop in a little seaside town so I could indulge in a panic purchase of Fruit Salad sweets, because I just *had* to have them.

In the final afternoon in our rental cottage, I walked downstairs to my dad catching up on the news. He asked, 'Where was it you thought you were going in April?'

'Venice. Why?' I replied.

'Doesn't look like you are, sweetheart.'

As I sat there, staring at the television, open mouthed and in utter bewilderment, I don't think I had any real grasp on just how much our lives were about to change in the coming weeks. We were watching scenes from Venice, live on TV, almost a ghost town – shut down by the police because of a virus. A virus that all of us would be in some way touched by over the next months, a world pandemic, in fact. Covid-19.

As we drove back home that day, it was all we heard on the news. Everyone was panic stricken. The nightly news reported death toll numbers like sports scores from countries in all corners of the globe. What on earth was happening? It felt as though something strange was on the horizon, for all of us. Something huge.

A couple of days later, I made it to my parents' house for my mum's birthday, completely oblivious to the fact that it would be the last time I saw them for months. The following day, Nico accompanied me to our next scan at the hospital and a check-up with our consultant, just as we had done in previous appointments. He was running late as his train was delayed so I decided to meet him at the hospital as I didn't want to risk being late too. It took every ounce of determination I had to walk into that scan room alone, dreading what today's news might be. Too terrified to look at the screens I lay there looking at my phone screen instead, desperately hoping Nico would call or tell me how close he was. The sonographer said, 'I can wait a few more minutes but then I need to bring my next lady in.'

She busily continued clicking away, scanning spine and head, heart chambers and kidneys. Everything in the most careful detail. A few moments later, my husband came bursting through the door, accompanied by one of the nurses who knew us from the EPU. He looked completely flustered but was just in time to see a heartbeat and a baby wriggling and for us to both to know that the baby was still doing just fine. I am so glad he made it, as we didn't know that day but it would be the last scan he was allowed to come along to for the entire duration of this pregnancy. Within a week or two he wouldn't even be travelling into London and not long after that our entire country would be shut down, too. We left that day clutching another precious scan photo and completely oblivious to what still lay ahead.

What unfolded in the coming weeks was beyond anything I could have comprehended, certainly at a time when we were finally expecting our rainbow baby, after all this time.

'Trust me,' I said to my mum on the phone, 'to finally get pregnant again, and in the middle of a fucking world pandemic.' We both laughed, we had to. It was certainly a laugh or you'll cry (again) moment; you just couldn't make it up! It was beyond surreal. Schools and shops closing all around, the government performing daily news conferences complete with panels of scientists and graphs to accompany statistics of rising infections and deaths, and then complete shutdown. I am certain we will all look back on that time and wonder what happened, why and how it seemed to propel itself with such force, so quickly and tear through the heart of not just our little island but the entire globe. It was nothing short of terrifying.

My worries of being pregnant again paled into insignificance when compared to what some families were having to face. Doctors and nurses fighting a daily battle against an invisible enemy, set to take down anyone in its path. It all seemed like a horrible nightmare, like watching a disaster movie unfolding in front of your eyes, except realising you're watching the news and that Tom Cruise isn't about to swoop in and save us all.

I was crippled with fear of leaving the house for the first few days after everything shut down. Pregnant women had been announced as 'vulnerable'. I didn't know what that meant, or *why*, but it scared the absolute shit out of me. This baby, this pregnancy, everything that had led up to this moment had seemed like such a marathon, and now *this*? What would happen if I got poorly? So many questions were on a constant loop around my head, again.

It was only a few days before I had to venture into hospital, but alone this time. It felt spooky. No throngs of people in the cafés or main entrance hall. I was greeted by a security guard wearing a mask at the main door. My appointment was checked and I was permitted to enter. As I walked slowly around to the obstetrics outpatients department, I became aware of the difference in atmosphere. Staff wearing masks; no one but medical staff in the little M&S that would ordinarily be bustling with people. I was next greeted by another member of staff, this time a nurse, wearing a mask, gloves and an apron. Ready to take my temperature before I entered the outpatient department. I was asked to sanitise my hands and take a seat. There were no other people waiting in this usually packed-out corridor. So many times I had sat and waited here, for good news and for bad. So many times, I had been triggered by happy-go-lucky bump-rubbing mamas-to-be as I sat weeping into another leaflet or waiting to sign another set of pre-operative paperwork, while wanting to run from the building screaming. But for now, it was just me and my little bump, alone.

This place had become so familiar but today it felt completely alien. It wasn't long before I was called in by my consultant, who was wearing a mask and gloves too. She knew how nervous I was. I mean, she knew how bad this was for me under normal circumstances, let alone with this new worry to contend with too. So she agreed to let me FaceTime Nico while she did the scan, as these *really were* extenuating circumstances. My scan double-checked every millimetre of this baby. She clicked through: brain, heart, kidneys, length of baby's legs . . . The list went on. All the while I stared at the screen, scrutinising every measurement. My heart skipping a beat every time she lingered a little too long over a certain area or stopped to double-check something. Each time, I was always convinced that this would be the time something was wrong. There was no ignorant bliss, rather a perpetual state of fear. I preferred to watch my husband's face on the phone screen instead, his

reaction and smile at every glimpse of the baby filled
me with joy.

'Baby is doing well. All developing well and normal
and healthy at this stage.'

'Thank you.' I always thanked her each time. I felt
as though it was the least I could do. She had been so
instrumental in getting us to this point and was doing
so much to look after us. I expect she couldn't quite
believe that a pandemic had been thrown into the
mix either. But baby was safe and well, normal and
healthy. That was all we could hope for.

The plan had originally been that I would have
scans every four weeks from twelve weeks, and then
every two as D-day drew closer. We were more than
halfway through and already that was turned on its
head. The hospital were trying to limit the number
of people who came in, quite rightly, and so my
next scan would need to wait for another six weeks.
I didn't know how I could wait that long. Silly, I
know, considering with most pregnancies you don't
get to see much of the baby (if at all) after 20 weeks.
But those scans had proved a lifeline so far. If we
could see the baby, know that everything was OK
for now and get to ride that blissful high if only
just for one day, then it would be enough to see me

through at least a week before the panic began to creep in.

Instead, the next few weeks of waiting would be interspersed with a midwife appointment and a doppler to listen in (which she would let me film so I could play it back when I needed to ease my anxiety). By the end of four weeks, I was climbing the walls again, ready to see that baby on the screen and to be told everything was still OK. Four weeks felt like my upper limit, but there wasn't a choice, it would be six at the earliest.

It wasn't just the prospect of not being able to access the additional medical support as often as we had planned for, it was that every other line of support had gone too. Everything I had used to cope over the last four years since Teddy died had seemingly vanished overnight. Yoga classes were cancelled; instead we were thrust into the online world of at-home classes where it was all I could do to ignore the pug barking at the birds in the garden or the kids in the garden next door sounding as if they were set to kill one another. My husband would be stepping over me to get to the coffee machine as I attempted down-dog in the middle of the kitchen. It wasn't long before I gave up and opted for a quiet 20-minute practice here and there, on my own, at quiet times and away from the glare of a laptop screen.

My regular acupuncture and therapy seemed a distant memory too – all of the tools I had become so reliant on to keep my fractious mind from over-thinking and to enable me to manage my grief had gone in a flash. These were such minor things in the grand scheme of things; everyone had their worries and things to deal with. Nico and I were lucky we were both still able to work and that was a blessing and something we had to be truly thankful for. We were also incredibly lucky that none of our family were frontline workers and that everyone, for now, was seemingly safe and well.

It was around this time, April 2020, that I reverted to a tactic I had used not long after Teddy died to get me through the harder days. I would repeat to myself over and over all of the things we'd had and all of the things that we were so lucky to still have. I found this got me through the harder days, the days I was missing a hug from my mum or a long-overdue catch up with a friend. The days when I felt scared for this baby and what the future might hold. I decided to say to myself, *We get to be safe at home* rather than *We are stuck at home*. I found that this helped, a little.

It was around this time I decided that I was ready to tell everyone our happy news. Everything seemed so heavy in the world right now and it was a dark and scary place for so many. I had wondered, often, how I would ever say anything on Instagram or my blog for fear of upsetting anyone else who was struggling, especially now, what with the pandemic having such a deep and frightening impact on people's lives. I was all too aware of the number of friends who had had IVF cycles cancelled, some after weeks of preparations and medications, others literally days away from embryo transfer. Our news, although wonderful for us, seemed such unfair timing for so many. On the one hand, I was eternally grateful that we had been so lucky; on the other, I had a serious bout of 'survivor's guilt' that was weighing heavily around my neck. I felt as though I didn't deserve such happiness when so many people were having a bloody awful time. The last thing I wanted to do was cause anyone else upset.

I thought long and hard about how I would tell the world our news on social media and I decided to ask my friend Anna, an artist who goes by the name of Sketchy Muma, to create a picture for me that would say it better than I ever could with words. She did the most perfect job and it was beyond anything I could have wished for. A simple sketch of us, with Boris at our feet, a rainbow on my tummy, and a little star in the sky with a T inside it. Above us were the words, 'Sometimes it takes so much courage to hope, but hope we did.'

It said everything it needed to say and people who weren't in a place to be able to hear the news would know they might not want to read the caption but I hoped that it was done delicately and sensitively enough so as not to trigger anyone in that moment. I knew, too well, what these posts had done to me in the past. How scan photos and cradled bumps would have me wanting to throw my phone out of the window. That lurch in my stomach as I told myself again and again *I'm happy for them, I'm just sad for us*, repeated over like some kind of infertility mantra. I knew there would be people who would feel that however I decided to tell them. I accompanied it with a caption that I thought about for a long time, something I had written over and over, writing and deleting, correcting as I dipped into the notes section on my phone where it had been saved. How could I explain to people how happy we were but how fearful we still were for the journey that lay ahead of us?

Eventually, I decided upon this:

Always believe . . .

Over five and a half years ago we began trying for a baby. Almost four years have passed since we held Teddy in our arms and then had to say good-bye. Three more babies lost since. Three years of fertility treatment. Three rounds of IVF.

So many tears.

BUT, sometimes magic can happen when you are waiting . . . . . .

I've wondered whether to share this news at all. I've battled to get through each day; each appointment, each scan, each reaction from the people we have told. My anxiety is beyond anything I can articulate, especially with everything going on in the world right now. The truth is, we are SO happy and hopeful, but terrified and still heartbroken, all rolled into one.

We've made it to a point that it finally felt right to share it with you too. So I wanted to do that through the genius that is my dear friend @sketchymuma.

We hope to bring Teddy's little brother or sister home this summer.

#teddyisgoingtobeabigbrother #believeinmagic #rainbowbaby #atlast

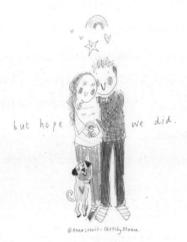

Sometimes it takes so much courage to hope,

but hope we did.

©Anna Lewis - Sketchy Munra

There were the obligatory emojis of rainbows and stars thrown in for Instagram readability!

I hoped it did the job. I had never been so scared to post anything before; my heart was pounding and I was shaking before I pressed *share*. This was it. People would finally know, after months of hiding, that we were at last set to become parents again. It hadn't been easy and, for now, it would continue that way, because everything had changed and we were in the middle of a global pandemic to boot . . .

Chapter 18

'It'll Be *Fine* This Time'

(and other things not to say)

'SO, HOW ARE YOU FEELING?'

The inevitable question, the answer to which sits just on the tip of my tongue and yet seems almost impossible to propel out into the universe. The answer was so complex, so multi-layered and, most likely, quite scary for most to have to be on the receiving end of, that more often than not I replied with something far easier, far more palatable for the recipient. I have found the answer to this question impossible to articulate fully or clearly. There were thoughts so dark, so scary, that I still daren't take myself back to that place for fear of falling down that black hole again.

Most of the time, I tried my best to keep myself in a positive space. One that wasn't consumed by thoughts of *Will my baby die, again?* or *What if my baby has already died and I just don't know yet?* Instead, I attempted to replace them with affirmations like: *Different pregnancy, different outcome.* I'll admit that this was definitely some last-ditch attempt by me to trick my subconscious into a false (and temporary) sense of security, to stop my thoughts trailing off to those darker places. It's a well-practised form of self-preservation; not to think about things too much, while also trying to remain in a positive mind-frame.

I am still pregnant, the baby is still doing well and things will be different, this time. I repeated this to myself on a loop. But truth be told? It was pretty fucking exhausting. It's mind-blowing how being caught in the ups and downs of your own head all day can completely wipe you out. To the point where, when someone does ask that dreaded question, 'How are you feeling?', you find yourself trying to answer, but absolutely no sound comes out at all.

I know that people's intentions were kind and genuine, that they wanted to check up on me, see how I was doing and ultimately how I was coping with another pregnancy. I always kept that in mind, that they cared enough to ask in the first place. I wish I could have answered, I really do, but most of the time it was all I could do to get through each day/hour/minute of those feelings myself without getting completely lost in them. It was as if I was just about peeking up out of the water, gasping for air and hoping nothing dreadful pulled me back under. When you are fighting that hard, kicking your legs that much to just stay afloat, sometimes you just don't have any energy left to answer that question and give any more energy to the situation. I don't want to be dismissive of people's concern for me but at the same time I was just not able to give any energy to explaining the complexities of my emotions. It's a situation that will, no doubt, have them walking away feeling better about everything, but leave me feeling more exhausted and wrung-out than ever about those worries and fears. Plus, an honest answer, one that touched on my deepest anxieties about carrying another baby and the potential of actually getting to the point where I gave birth again, was so often met with . . .

'Well, you really must try not to worry so much. Just try to relax and enjoy it.'

This response had me wishing I had never trusted to let that person a little way into those deep worries at all. If only it was that easy, hey? Just try not to worry! I'm a positive person, I always have been a glass half-full kind of girl – I am pretty sure to the point of irritation for most people. So, it seems impossible for me to fathom that anyone would have thought that I *wasn't* trying not to worry, trying my very fucking best just to get through each day and not completely lose my mental shit to that gaping chasm of terrifying emotions. No part of me ever wanted to feel like this, to worry that much or to lie awake at night playing out every single possible scenario simply so that I could feel 'prepared' for the worst to happen.

I spent a lot of my time just wanting to feel normal again (whatever that was!), and I wished, every day, that losing Teddy hadn't robbed me of that pure joy and happiness that any expectant mother should be entitled to, but it did. Even the affirmations, the yoga, the long walks and the 'switching off' couldn't save me from my own thoughts when they started to take hold. So when someone said something as simple and dismissive as 'It'll be fine this time' or 'I've got a good feeling', it only added to the pressure that my thoughts were unjustified somehow, that I was not perfectly within my rights to be feeling them after my son died.

I 'had a good feeling' before Teddy was born, a bloody good feeling, and I was so excited to be a mum, but he died. So, I know that no amount of good feelings (and/or vibes) will change the outcome of any subsequent pregnancy or birth; it really is a lottery of life where anything can happen and we are all simply at the mercy of the universe and what it has decided to deliver to us in that given moment. It might be wonderful but, as I already knew, it might be impossibly shit; something that could shift your entire world on its axis and never allow you to 'just believe' or 'try not to worry' again.

See, I warned you it was a complex answer.

Another few 'wise words' I found particularly hard to digest came from someone on the internet when I posted about my inability to answer the 'question' about feelings in the later stages of pregnancy after loss. Now, I must warn you here, that my first ever teacher at college told me if I wanted to pursue my chosen career at the time then I 'must never talk about religion or politics with clients' and, well, I am about to break that golden rule now, so look away if you're likely to be upset or offended.

A woman wrote to me: 'I'm telling you to put all of your faith in Jesus.' Um, no thank you, I'm fine. Jokes aside, it made me feel as though she really thought I wasn't trying hard enough, as if I wasn't putting my own energy/thoughts/wishes into something that I believed in. As if I wasn't doing enough for our baby to ensure it all went well. I'm all for believing in whatever you want to believe in – absolutely, each to their own and I pass zero judgement on anyone from any faith who uses that faith to support themselves in their lives and their own personal journey. I just felt that telling a bereaved mother (who wasn't a close friend or a family member, or actually someone you had ever met) to trust in something/someone that had no bearing or impact on her life in order to 'guarantee' a much happier outcome was, well, quite frankly, just a little bit insensitive.

It's a tough one, as I know subjects like that can be contentious and divisive and, as someone who doesn't believe in any (of the many) gods, I'm probably (read: definitely) not the best person to address the subject. I do know what it feels like to have your world turned on that axis though, to lose a child and to know that no matter how much you had hoped/prayed/wished for a different outcome, that it still would have been the same. That's when I feel like comments like that, however well meaning, must go unsaid, or at least be aimed at someone you know well enough and who shares the same beliefs as you. Pregnancy after loss is hard enough without being told to take up a new faith while you're at it.

It goes without saying that the 'try not to worry'/'it will be fine' gang are almost always (always) people who have themselves never experienced anything less than a straightforward or happy pregnancy. Their comments come from a place of positivity, a naivety that has long since left my mind and it's something that I am incredibly envious of. Although sometimes I do fear that this kind of 'toxic positivity' can often be more damaging than supportive. I'm not mad at them, nor do I want to dismiss their genuine concern about how I might be feeling on any given day. It's just a tough pill to swallow when your pregnancy is caught up with so many complex worries – culminating in a crippling anxiety that you will, yet again, leave the hospital empty-armed with an empty car seat in the back of the car – and someone says, 'It'll be fine.'

So what do I feel would have been a better response? I suppose I was simply longing for them to say to me in that moment something along the lines of: 'You're right, it must be unimaginable for you to get through each day worrying that the same thing might happen again. It's shit, and I wish you didn't have to feel this way. I hope you know that everyone is rooting for the best outcome for you and that everything you are feeling is normal. Just try to get through each day, each hour if you have to; that's all you can do, and I am here if you ever do want to talk about it.'

In short: *I can't understand, I'll never 'get it', but I'm here and I hope you're OK*. I'm unsure if anyone who's experiencing a worrying pregnancy, or a pregnancy after loss, wants to be fed false platitudes or needs someone to just tell them 'I've got a good feeling.' It merely undermines those (valid) emotions they are feeling and most likely makes them feel even more guilty about feeling them.

Guilt, that's another thing. With all of the worries and the anxiety, then comes the guilt. The guilt that I didn't feel happy every moment of every day in this pregnancy, like I did in my first. I felt guilty that I was carrying this baby every day and worrying that it will die, rather than being excited for his or her arrival. Guilty that I didn't feel excited, like I should have done, like society tells us we should be, especially when we longed for it so badly.

I was trying to explain it to a friend not long after my 20-week scan and the only analogy I could come up with as to why my mind might be so convinced something would go wrong, was this: Imagine if every time you got in your car to drive somewhere you crashed. Every time. It didn't matter where your starting point was, or where you were going, it just happened again. You changed your car and you still crashed. You began to become scared that each time you tried again, it would happen again. All the while you watched as your friends jumped in their cars and seamlessly cruised from A to B, always arriving safely at their destination and in a timely fashion. Why couldn't that happen for you? When would that happen for you? Surely you would only ever feel like it wouldn't happen when, one day, you got in the car, drove safely from A to B and nothing went wrong? Then, and only then, could you start to believe the next time you got in the car and set off on a journey that the outcome would be a good one.

That was how I saw this pregnancy. Teddy had died, we had then lost three more babies over two consecutive pregnancies thereafter. In my mind, this could also end in disaster and no amount of positive thinking would help me to see a way past that. The only thing that would change my pattern of thinking and allow my subconscious to believe that it didn't always go wrong would be to successfully complete a healthy pregnancy and leave the hospital with a living, breathing baby. Thus, getting from A to B, safely. Then, maybe next time (if there ever is a next time), I wouldn't feel this way. Perhaps each subsequent pregnancy after loss would get easier? I am yet to discover that, and perhaps I never will.

I remember my friend nodding in agreement. She hadn't ever experienced the loss of a baby but this made it make sense. Why wouldn't I think something would go wrong if it always had before? It obviously wasn't a case of wanting it to, nor willing it to, or even being unable to 'think positively'. It was simply past trauma, lived experience, that leads your mind to thinking a certain thing is bound to happen, no matter how much you don't want it to.

I hoped that if I could just make it through each day and get safely to the end of this pregnancy, I could retrain my brain to believe that good things can happen. It was more a case of surviving than thriving in this pregnancy, which sounds sad, but it was the truth.

As for the guilt? That was something I would have to continue to manage too. I knew I loved this baby beyond measure. I didn't actually think it would be possible for a baby to be more loved or longed-for than this one. We wanted this little one in our lives so much. Not only because we had been so ready to be parents when Teddy had arrived four years before but because subsequently our love and parental emotions had, at times, felt as if they had no place to go. There had been no little person here to channel all of that love and energy into, so we had had to find alternatives, such as fundraising, writing and keeping our parental journey alive. But that was all about to change, and this baby, whoever they might turn out to be, would be everything we had wished for. If only they knew how loved they already were; we hoped (every day) that they would arrive safely to be able to feel that love. So, despite the guilt, the trauma, the anxiety and all of the other emotions piled in on top of that, we knew this baby would be loved, and that our love for our baby was not related to the answer of the dreaded 'How are you feeling?' question, however difficult that was to explain.

It's not that I wanted anyone to be scared to ask that question, I just wanted people to be prepared for the answer because ultimately it might be one that they didn't want, or weren't prepared, to hear.

When there is any level of complex emotion involved with someone's current situation, whether grieving or navigating a difficult personal situation, if you ask them how they are feeling then you have to want to listen to the answer if they are willing (and able that day) to give it. You have to truly want to know and not just be asking because it makes you feel better or gives you the feeling that you've 'done the right thing'. If someone asked me then they had to be prepared for me to tell them about my anxiety and the fear that was eating me up daily. They needed to acknowledge that and not greet it with a dismissive, 'Oh, it will be fine.' Because then I ended up wishing I hadn't given them that piece of my heart, as it appeared to me that they didn't really care for the answer in the first place. They just wanted to hear, 'Yeah, I'm fine.' Which was, of course, a lie, but one I found myself feeding to people so often in order to make them feel better for having asked, and as a way of me avoiding a way of facing those feelings.

Sometimes I found myself saying something along the lines of: 'Yep, feeling fine physically, it's just the emotional side that's a bit too complex to explain.' I hoped this would indicate to whoever had asked that I just couldn't face talking about it that day. Those were usually the days on which feelings had already exhausted me to the point of desperation and I just couldn't face making anyone feel better by pretending

I was fine. The truth is, unless you have a fully functioning crystal ball (in which case I am most definitely in the market and very interested in where I can get my hands on one of those), then none of us really know that everything will be fine. We can only hope that it will be and we cling to that hope, every day, with all our might.

Chapter 19

Holding on to Hope

HOPE IS SOMETHING I HAVE TALKED ABOUT, AND WRITTEN ABOUT, *A LOT*. Being pregnant again during a global pandemic, while being cut off physically from our friends and family, meant hope became more than ever something we relied on. As we made it through the first month or so of our locked-down life, and my blossoming bump became impossible to hide as I approached the third trimester, we hoped for a lot of things. We hoped that we'd get a hug from our parents soon and that by the time this baby arrived things would resemble some kind of 'normal'. We still hoped that this baby would arrive safely and that no complications would arise between now and us coming home together.

I began to live week to week, but usually day to day and, sometimes, on the hardest days, hour to hour. Midwife appointments and consultant scans were the only major events in my diary. My husband was working from home, which was a huge comfort in itself. With a pregnancy that was so filled with worry and uncertainty, it felt nice to have one aspect of our lives that had improved: more time together. I began immersing myself in writing and, while the rest of the world was working out at 9am daily with Joe Wicks, perfecting their banana bread and prepping for yet another Zoom quiz/drinks night, I found myself wishing those weeks away.

Nothing felt more difficult than being apart from my mum. She had been with me through everything, through some of the very worst parts, and now I needed her through this, even if just for a coffee and a hug. I know technology is incredible and it keeps us connected but sometimes (most of the time) nothing can beat a *real* hug. We were living in a time when not even the midwives could hug me as I sat there sobbing and I could tell it went against the very nature of everything they had ever been taught and naturally wanted to do when supporting an expectant mother. Every conversation with anyone there to support us was had behind the cover of masks, leaving me unable to read the expressions of those who were there to help. I attended every appointment alone, staring at scan screens and desperately hoping that there wouldn't be any bad news.

During this time, I had contact from so many women through my blog and my Instagram who had lost a baby during lockdown. Their pain was unimaginable to me. I couldn't comprehend what it must be like to lose your child and not be immediately surrounded by your loved ones. I tried to imagine how different Teddy dying in those circumstances would have been but I couldn't even allow my mind to go there. There were mothers saying goodbye to their babies, on their own, no hug from friends and family, sometimes without their birth partner. It all seemed too painful and another place I couldn't allow my anxious mind to travel if I were to make it to the end of this pregnancy with my sanity intact. I knew, all too well, that awful things happen every day but for the moment I needed to guard my own heart and try to use this time away from normal life to stay protected in our little bubble.

I tried my hardest to focus on the positive things that we could do during this time. Ways we could prepare for this baby to arrive safely and will the universe to deliver that wish for us. We had most baby things from when we had been waiting for Teddy. All of the 'big stuff', as I would call it, had been packed safely away in the loft ever since the week after we had returned home from hospital in May 2016. I knew there would come a time when we needed to address it, do a full stocktake on what we had and see if there was anything we still needed. Plus, so much had changed in the four years since. Actually, everything seemed different.

The nursery, for the most part, had remained the same. The same furniture and sheepskin rug that had always felt heavenly between my toes, the same toys in the cot and the same mobile hanging from the ceiling that I had lovingly stitched in the weeks before Teddy arrived. It had been used on and off as a storage room during renovations, with boxes and stuff piled everywhere, but for now it was relatively clear and just needed a bit of an update. We both agreed it was a good idea to make some little changes in there, to freshen it up. To make it actually feel like we were nesting, properly, for *this* baby. I didn't want it to be as though we were bringing this precious baby home to a room we had prepared for their big brother. I'm sure that, had Teddy been here, we would have prepared a new room for this little one, so it should be no different. We decided to refresh the paint and change the shelves. I put up a new mirror in the shape of a rattan sunshine, replacing the old white one. We added little golden stars as wall stickers, hanging rainbows and new prints in frames above the cot. Little changes that made a huge difference to this tiny room.

I started collecting new clothes. I wanted this baby to have their *own* clothes that I had chosen just for them, I didn't want them to live in hand-me-downs from their big brother (albeit ones that had never actually left the drawer or been worn), I wanted them to have their own things. It became really important to me to do these little things as a positive step and I began, slowly, to really enjoy doing them. I actually felt *excited*. Doing the things that I had feared the most actually began to ignite that spark of excitement in me – that this might really be happening for us.

Of course, there was the fear still hanging in there and often influencing my purchasing decisions when researching anything we still needed. I found myself Googling 'safe sleep for babies', looking at mattress safety ratings, replacing the Moses basket mattress with one I deemed safer, and then deciding that the Moses basket would be used only for daytime naps and buying a new bedside crib on which the sides came down so I could be as physically close to this baby at all times, especially during the night. Getting through each night with a baby was something else that panicked me. Teddy had stopped breathing that first night he lay next to me sleeping in hospital. Surely I would never sleep again if another baby was sleeping next to me? I would be checking its breathing at every opportunity, watching this child sleep until it was at least 18. I lost myself in a world of baby sleep safety monitors and their reviews online, eventually settling on something called a Smartsock that was a little hospital-style bandage sock that strapped around the baby's foot and monitored its breathing and oxygen levels. It also linked to an app in your phone and had a whacking great alarm attached to it that was set to go off if things weren't being picked up. I knew it was extreme (as well as not being the cheapest option) but I just felt as though nothing would buy us the peace of mind we craved, so I may as well give this a shot.

We had a pram, a car seat and everything we would need to travel anywhere safely but we both agreed that these final elements would stay firmly in the loft until such a time that we were certain this baby had arrived and we had a time to come home. I couldn't face seeing my husband bringing that empty car seat back into the house again and having to stash it away out of sight, thinking I couldn't see him, all the while knowing his heart hurt as much as mine did. Buying the little bits and bobs, though, gave me the light relief I needed in between those heavier thoughts. I was building up quite the little collection of extra things for our special rainbow's arrival.

How I looked and felt physically now left no possible doubt that this was indeed happening. I was getting big, much bigger than I had ever been with Teddy. This baby was doing its best to let me know that it was alive and well in my tummy, mainly by kicking the shit out of me on a daily basis. Like Thumper the rabbit, they were crashing around in there, all the while unknowingly reassuring me that everything *would* be OK. No matter how big I was getting, I decided not to buy too many maternity clothes this time, instead opting for my usual style of dresses or tops in bigger sizes – I didn't want to make the mistake I had made when pregnant with Teddy of spending money on maternity clothes that never saw the light of day again after his arrival, while all of my pre-pregnancy clothes I could no longer fit so much as a big toe into, so I had to waste even more money on clothes to wear in the 'in-between' phase after birth. All of which I later came to hate and could never look at again because they reminded me of how sad I had felt. The end result was that the maternity clothes and in-between clothes ended up going to the charity shop following about three subsequent clear-outs that spanned a six-month aftermath period of me trying to be less of a miserable bastard and go back to wearing clothes that I enjoyed wearing again.

Well, not this time! I wouldn't be caught out and I wouldn't be wasting money on clothes I couldn't wear and enjoy after pregnancy. There is something to be said for being heavily pregnant in the spring/summer months, however hot and uncomfortable it may be. It made floaty dress upon floaty dress a viable wardrobe selection, most of which could be chosen with the goal of easy boob access for subsequent breastfeeding in mind. I hoped that these would all be things I wore in pregnancy and beyond, plus they made me happy and any extra sprinkling of joy right now was a blessing. Sometimes the lockdown bubble of floaty dresses, baby prep and internet shopping wasn't actually that bad at all; in fact, it felt a very safe bubble in which to exist.

Another thing that became increasingly difficult to consider was the packing of a hospital bag for the arrival of this baby. Perhaps it was because the last one had been packed with such joyous anticipation for our little bundle to arrive and things felt, well, just a little scarier this time? Or perhaps it was because the memory of unpacking that bag again and all of the tiny, clean, white clothes, all un-worn that were placed carefully back into drawers that would go un-touched for many years, was still one that haunted me. I remember the day I finally felt ready to go back into the nursery and unpack that bag that had been so lovingly and excitably packed by a heavily preg-nant me in 2016. It took me a couple of months be-fore I could even so much as look at it. So much so, that I had forgotten what I had packed, and seeing each item made my heart break all over again. I closed the drawers and didn't look again, so everything had stayed the same. That was, of course, until I began to collect things for this baby.

I didn't feel ready to pack a bag, not at the start of the third trimester, not at 35 weeks, as so many books and forums suggest (*after all, it could be any day now and you'll want to be prepared!*). Even the week before our scheduled arrival date it seemed like an impossible task to pack that bag. I knew nothing could prepare me for what was about to happen; no matter how many sleepsuits, fancy new maternity nighties or snacks and drinks I packed, all I wanted to prepare for was a living, breathing baby. All of the 'nice to haves' and the Mummy bloggers giving hints and tips of what to pack made me want to crawl under my duvet and only come out when it was all over.

What I found even more mind-blowing were the people who seemed to forget I had done it all before. It was as though because I didn't have Teddy here, people had erased the memory that I was already well versed in this preparation malarkey. People started sending me tips of what to pack for hospital and things to remember. To which I usually responded, 'Yes, I did that last time,' with an emphasis on the *last time*. It made me think that many people still viewed me as a first-time mum, as if this was a first-time pregnancy, an entirely new experience.

Well, it was kind of an entirely new experience, and by that I mean one that they had no experience of. A pregnancy that was not filled with lists of what to pack and gender reveal cannons but rather one where my mind asked every day, 'Why pack a bag when your baby might not need anything?' We knew we were having a scheduled C-section and so, with that in mind, I just decided the easiest thing to do would be to pack my bags the night before, if we made it to that point without any action starting. That way, I could start collecting any bits and bobs I thought I might desperately need, but a fully packed bag wouldn't be sat there staring at me, a glaring reminder of the last one.

Friends also began to ask me questions about what we had/needed/hadn't bought yet. A couple asked what pram I would be buying. My response, 'The one in the loft that's been packed away for four years,' usually met with a message of 'Oh, of course'. I was using our same pram, just like they had done for their second, third and fourth children. The only difference was ours was still brand new, no wear and tear, and no time for me to have assessed whether it was practical and/or the right one for us. From that perspective I most certainly *was* a new mum; I hadn't had the chance to road-test any of the gear we had bought years ago. I didn't know what would work and what wouldn't, what was worth the money and what would prove to be a total waste. We were rookies, in that sense.

I had put two nappies on Teddy during his entire three days on this earth. One the day he was born and the second just before we changed him into clothes again before he died. I was a novice at wrangling new-born babies into clothes or swaddles and that thought terrified me too. This little baby would be so precious; I didn't want to fuck it up this time and get anything wrong. But I suppose that's a worry all new parents have and I just had to accept that there would be things that we would get wrong. That we'd just be learning as we went.

All in all, during a global pandemic, you're pretty protected from most things if you spend your entire life at home as we did. I was completely shielded from all of the questions that strangers, people in shops might ask me: 'Is it your first?' or 'So, do you know what you're having?' Total strangers speculating on the contents of my womb, all because I was sporting a bump. I had become accustomed to these sorts of questions while heavily pregnant with Teddy and the answers would roll off my tongue with ease (yes and no). This time though, there weren't any strangers to bump into because when I did go out to walk Boris (my government-approved daily exercise) there was simply no one around and, even if there was, everyone was far too busy keeping their distance from one another. I don't think I realised how lucky this made me during this pregnancy until such a time when I was catapulted back into situations where those questions might arise – and they did, quite unprovoked, in fact.

As summer progressed and lockdown started to ease a little, we were free to begin doing little 'normal' things once more. We found ourselves in a local town one Sunday morning before heading out on a walk with Boris. We picked up a takeaway iced coffee and queued for buns from the bakery. As we all stood a safe two metres apart, queuing along the pavement waiting for the bakers, I noticed a couple of women around my age in front of us in the queue, obviously there picking up supplies for a park picnic together. They were excitedly chatting and waiting for a third friend who appeared a few moments later to join them; they squealed with delight as she approached, her twin babies stacked in a rather fancy looking pram and they all proceeded to coo over them. It was at this point one of them went in and the other stayed out on the pavement to wait with the new mum and her babies. As we drew closer to the door, the mum who had arrived seemed to clock me out of all the 20-or-so people standing in the queue and almost shouted to me, 'When are you due?'

None of your business, total stranger, was the obvious answer that sprung to mind (forgive me for not being overly friendly but I was panic stricken by the direct nature of her unexpected question and really aware that I had an audience of over 20 people now standing behind me, who were no doubt as bored as I was in that queue and now listening for my answer).

I hesitated. 'Next month,' I said, not wanting to give any shred of detail.

'Is it your first?' she continued.

Fuck. *How am I going to get out of this one?* I felt my stomach lurch and my mouth become dry with nerves. Fuck it, I'm going in . . .

'No, no it's not,' I replied.

She paused as she looked at us and down at our legs only to be greeted with the sight of a confused and rather hot-looking pug. She continued, looking a little confused herself. 'Your second?'

'Yes, our second,' I confirmed.

'Ah, lovely,' she said as she looked even more confused and returned to her chat with friends.

Maybe she thought our other little one was with grandparents or friends? Or perhaps she feared what the answer might be if she continued her questioning? I'll never know as the conversation stopped dead there, as did my happy, care-free mood that day. Those questions would always be there, waiting to jump out at me when I least expected them; to catch me unaware and remind me that I might have to reveal my most painful life experience to a total stranger at any given moment. I wasn't about to deny Teddy's existence, he *was* my first, and this child would be our second.

'What would you have done if she'd carried on?' asked my husband as we walked back around the corner, away from the bakers and laden with buns. 'If she'd asked where our other child was?'

'I'd have answered her honestly. Said that he should have been just four but that he died as a baby. Pretty sure that would have capped off the conversation just as quickly.'

He shook his head and laughed.

I don't want to live in fear of being able to mention Teddy. I almost hoped she had asked that next question as I wondered what her reaction might have been. Would it have stopped her ever asking a stranger questions like that again? Would others in the queue have gasped in horror and wanted the ground to swallow them whole as the awkwardness washed over everyone in sight? I'll never know but it did make me appreciate just how sheltered we had been from conversations like that while hiding in our own homes, baking for 12 weeks. Perhaps the lockdown had actually done me a huge favour?

This experience also made me think about how I would handle those questions going forward and how I might answer them if we were finally lucky enough to bring a baby home. How many 'Is it your first?'s would there be? Would people recoil when I told them the truth or would they want to hear about this baby's big brother? We would have to wait and see. For now, I sipped my iced coffee and began to contemplate which bun I would eat first . . .

As the global state of affairs rumbled on, and things began to return to something almost recognisable as normal life (I mean, if you squinted *a lot*, and remembered to wear your mask!), our due date drew closer and my tummy grew ever bigger. I remember thinking, *we've got to a point where I can count the weeks' wait on one hand* – that felt like a milestone in itself. When I first saw those two lines appear back in early December, I never dared to dream we would make it this far and yet here we were.

As the date drew closer, my anxiety continued to grow with more vigour than ever before, becoming harder to manage. I had so many worries still swirling around my head. I knew we could guarantee a date and type of delivery (almost, if the baby stayed put as hoped for) but I couldn't be sure of anything that would happen next.

For us, that was when the trouble had started. Teddy had stopped breathing that first night in hospital; there was no way I could face a night, alone, on a hospital ward staring at a new-born baby and willing it to keep on breathing, but that was going to be the situation with current hospital guidelines as they were. No partners or husbands were allowed to stay; they could be there for delivery and a few hours after but no longer. That thought alone crippled me into a state of frozen panic. Surely none of the other new mums around me in that ward would be spending the night wondering if their baby was going to live or die? That image of Teddy being carried away played again and again. The lights flashing, people running down corridors and curtains swiftly being pulled around our hospital ward bay. How would I manage that if I had to face it alone?

I cried down the phone to the mental health midwife, expressing all of my worst fears and trying my best to get across to her that no matter how many people told me that things would be different this time, that was all that played out in my head. I could hear in her voice that she understood how fearful I was. She knew that no amount of positive thinking or difference in delivery would save me from being terrified that first night.

Fortunately, I think because it was deemed my mental health was a risk, the hospital agreed that I wouldn't have to stay alone overnight. Nico could stay too and have a Covid-19 test (as I would at my pre-operative appointment) and we would be put in a room away from those familiar wards that I feared so much. She also suggested it would be a good idea for me to visit before delivery, to walk around and see it all again before we found ourselves arriving to have this baby.

The trauma of walking out on the day Teddy was transferred to the neonatal intensive care unit lived with me, as did the feeling of leaving after delivering our next baby in 2017. It wasn't a place that held many happy memories for us, apart from the ones of bringing Teddy into the world, which were the happiest. I wanted to focus on those, on how it had felt that evening when we had first wheeled him from the delivery room to the ward in his little tank. How I had wanted to show him off to everyone I passed and tell them what I had made. That was the feeling I was working on for this little baby too, trying my best to channel that energy, that hope, into happy thoughts. Everyone was doing so much for us to make sure this baby was well looked after, and that my anxiety wouldn't get the better of me before D-day.

At one of my last scans with our consultant, I sat crying, again, after we had seen a perfectly healthy baby, growing well, on the screen. The 4D scan had allowed us to see the baby sucking its fingers and wrapping its other hand around the top of its face. Every detailed 4D photo she attempted to capture for us looked like a piece of modern art, something that wouldn't look out of place in the Tate, where people would stop and stare, wondering where hands ended and face began. Finally, she got a perfect picture of the baby's face, the first one she had managed to capture during the entire pregnancy. Their little squashed nose and rosebud lips, a hand cupped around its chin. In that moment, I felt as though I could have stared at that little face for an eternity, wondering *who* it was inside there.

The magical moment was suddenly burst with the onset of panic. This little person in there was so precious, the unsurmountable fear that I might lose them was too much to contemplate. Not the usual fears most mums-to-be have in the scanning room, I'm sure. I couldn't hide my emotions and, as I climbed off the bed and onto the chair to chat to my consultant about 'the plan', all of my fears began to spill out in one long blubbering stream. She must have wondered what on earth was going on at this point.

I couldn't face the prospect of delivering this baby on a Monday, which was the day that had been bandied about. Teddy was born on a Monday and died on a Thursday. Those days in between had been utter torment, I never wanted to re-live them; this needed to be different. I couldn't face an evening delivery either, not having a baby and going almost straight to sleep like last time. I needed this baby to be born in the morning. I wanted the opportunity to stare at them, all day (because that's what people do with new-borns, isn't it?!), and I didn't want to miss a second of that. Essentially, I needed *everything* to be different. It was as if taking control of these things would somehow give me more control of the situation and, ultimately, of the outcome. I knew nothing could change what was already written in the stars but I wanted to try my hardest to do the very best for that perfect little face I had just seen on the screen.

My consultant assured me that they would try to deliver the baby in the morning, that the only thing that would bump me down the list would be an emergency, which of course was beyond anyone's control. She also explained that, all being well, she would try to deliver the baby on the Thursday before but that it fell a day short of my 38-week mark and she didn't want to put this baby at any undue risk. They didn't plan for scheduled caesarean sections at the weekend, so the Friday or the Monday were the only options. For me, Friday was also a preference as it meant we would get to meet this baby sooner, a moment I was longing for. I wanted this worry to be over. I ached to hold this baby in my arms and know that he or she was OK. To hear a baby cry or see them open their eyes; two things we had never known before. I tried to play a new image over and over in my mind instead, one that hadn't actually happened yet; one that saw our consultant lifting this baby safely out into the world and hearing those first screaming cries fill the room. I focused all my energy during quiet times of reflection playing that in my mind, willing it to happen, imagining every detail of the room and how it would feel. It was doing things like that which enabled me to keep my mind focused on the hope that we had and not the fear that was trying to take hold.

As the days and weeks progressed, I found myself avoiding people more than ever. Willing the days to pass and mentally ticking them off as they did. I couldn't face being asked how I was, I just needed to get through it. Friends called and FaceTimed, all eagerly asking, 'Have you got a date yet?' When we finally did I knew couldn't share it, I was too scared. Most people seem to happily share their due date with anyone who will listen – I know I had last time around – but this became a closely guarded secret. Not only because of the worry that engulfed us both but because it wasn't an 'estimated due date'. It was, to all intents and purposes, an *actual* delivery date. Set in stone: the day we would finally meet this baby. I didn't want people holding their breath and staring at their phones the day it finally happened, I didn't want anyone to shoulder the worry of a safe arrival. That was ours to carry. I know that some people might feel happier, comforted, encouraged even by having more people know but it's personal preference and this was what felt right for us to get us to that date.

The days seemed to move in slow motion. June and July were baking, as you might expect. I didn't want to complain about the heat, even though I had several kilograms strapped to my front by this point and was melting most days. If someone had told me this time last year, as I lay just waking up from my last procedure with my consultant to remove that 'debris' (as it had so eloquently been labelled!), that I'd be weeks away from having another baby, I'd have hugged them forever. I remembered feeling so sad, so empty, last summer, when we were constantly chasing a dream of becoming parents again. As if we were crashing from cycle to cycle, procedure to treatment, all the while putting everything on hold while we held on to that finally becoming our reality. It had been so tiring, to say the least. So, I couldn't bring myself to complain, no matter how hot, how heavy, how scared I began to feel.

Because, finally, a dream was about to come true.

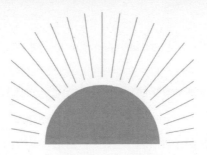

Chapter 20

It's All About You, Baby

THOSE LAST FEW WEEKS DIDN'T GET ANY EASIER (I'D *LOVE* TO START THIS CHAPTER ON A LIGHTER NOTE, BUT, YOU KNOW, HONESTY BEING THE BEST POLICY AND ALL THAT!). I checked my phone calendar each morning when I woke, counting days and feeling my anxiety mount. It felt like a bizarre cocktail of crippling worry and excited anticipation. I was so eager to meet whoever had been inhabiting my uterus for the last nine months but simultaneously terrified of losing them. That time was as night and day to how I had felt in the lead up to Teddy's birth and I spent much of the time longing for just a little flicker of that ignorant bliss to return.

My last scan with my consultant went much like the others: still alone, still wearing a medical face mask to the appointment that morning and still terrified of bad news. Once more, I watched the little person wriggling on the screen, arms and leg movements more definite than ever, tiny hands covering a squished-up face as if to say, '*Please, no more photos!*' My consultant reassured me (yet again) that she believed the baby was healthy and thriving in there. I watched the screen intently, for the last time, as she scanned every detail again and measured everything she could.

'OK, I'm happy. So, let's get a date booked in for delivery.'

In that moment, shit got extremely real. A date, an actual date. Something I had been plodding painfully towards for so many months was finally going to be in front of me. I sat and watched as she clicked through her diary on the computer screen, eventually calling through to the delivery suite to confirm the date and time for the delivery. It felt surreal, just booking in to have this baby. She handed me the paperwork and another bundle of scan photos and that was that. I clutched it all closely to my chest as I left the room, not quite believing that would be my final time in there with this baby inside me. As I thanked her, she turned in her chair and said, 'I'll see you then.' I joked in response, 'Yep, all I need to do is ask this little one to stay put for the two and a half weeks!' And with that, I was gone.

Walking out of the hospital felt final in some way, although I knew it wouldn't be at all as I'd be back in less than two weeks for my pre-operative injections. I think it was just knowing that that part of the journey was over: the certainty of scheduled scans, the knowing that there was always the next check – that next little slice of reassurance. We were coming to the end of the road and getting through this last part would be all down to me.

Now I knew the date I felt as though I was harbouring an even bigger secret from the world. Who should we even tell? The pressure felt immense. Not only because of the mounting fear we both had for those 72 hours that would follow the birth but because we both knew that we couldn't quite cope with that added pressure of people worrying about us in the lead up to an imminent arrival. After less than a minute of discussion, we decided it would be best to only tell our parents when the baby would be delivered; it felt safer that way. After all, they would be the people we would need around us if anything were to go wrong. I arranged for my parents to come to our house the day before to collect Boris and so that I could see them one final time before the day. My mum also came to visit the week before, to help me finally wash the clothes, muslins and other baby-related items that had sat in drawers or lay crisply untouched in new packets for fear of 'jinxing' the final furlong.

With a week to go, it did seem that the most sensible thing to do was to make some kind of effort with preparations. It was another baking hot July day and I watched on as my mum carefully pegged up tiny sleepsuits, hats and fresh muslins on the line. She was smiling as she did it, everything glinting perfectly in the afternoon sunshine as it billowed in the breeze. I remember feeling a sudden swell of emotion inside me, of love for the baby, for my mum and a real sense of how lucky we were to be in this position again. I knew my mum was excited, she was practically bristling with love and anticipation as she pegged up each little piece of clothing. I so wanted this, for her, as much as I did for myself. I even felt ready to lay some things out for my hospital bag that day. Doing these little things allowed it to feel ever so slightly more like I was beginning to manifest good energy and letting go of the fear a little. I knew that I had to allow the excitement to sit beside the fear, or the latter would take over.

I couldn't answer texts or calls from friends in those final days. It was as if women have a sixth sense for these things: I don't think my phone had ever run so red hot! Everyone seemed to be checking on me, sending sweet messages of, 'Thinking of you . . .' and 'Must not be long now . . .'

I showed my husband how many messages I had received in just one day from well-meaning friends who were checking in on me. 'Blimey, that's intense. You can't be having to answer everyone all of the time, you need to turn your phone off,' was his considered response. He was right. Well, to a certain extent. I wasn't about to turn my phone off (in case of emergency, haha!), but I did change my WhatsApp settings so that no one could see if I had been online or know if I had read their messages. It felt too much; if they knew I had read their message then I would feel obliged to reply and the obligation to do so would see me repeating the same well-practised response again and again, my anxiety mounting with each tap of the keyboard.

I had never been the kind of person who didn't want to hear from friends, who didn't love a good old catch-up or the opportunity to share my latest news in every inch of detail. This was an alien feeling. I wanted to run and hide. To curl up in a ball and go unnoticed by the world until this was all over. I wanted to try my best to explain, because I feel so passionately that the complexity of a pregnancy after loss is something we should all try to understand, but trying to do so when I was in the midst of those intense emotions just felt overwhelming. Other than talking to a couple of my closest friends, everything else went unanswered. I could tell them some news when I had some actual news to tell! Until then, I was in survival mode.

Just four days before what would be D-day, I was back at the hospital. This time in the maternity wing, for a pre-operative appointment and steroid injection. The injection needed to be administered in a certain timeframe before baby's arrival so that their lungs were 'ready' for the big wide world. There would be two injections, a day apart.

As I nervously pressed the buzzer to the doors of the maternity wing, I could feel my hands shaking. We had been for a brief tour of this part of the hospital with my mental health midwife just a few days after my final scan. Prior to that, the last time I had spent any time here was when I had delivered Teddy and our last baby. Those corridors were eerily familiar and I felt that same sense of panic beginning to rise in my chest. When I had been on the tour, I had had my husband by my side, ready to squeeze my hand, and me his, at any moment we needed it. But coming here alone felt different.

I walked towards the desk and looked through the glass windows into the wards. I remembered being in one of those rooms as I was being induced with Teddy. As I took each step along that corridor, it was as if I remembered everything and absolutely nothing about being there all at the same time; it was a blur. I tried my best to hold it together – I didn't want to cry today, I just wanted to get in and out and tick this next part off the list. After some confusion among the midwives about who I was and why I was there, and being asked at one point 'Is this your first baby?', to which the only answer I could muster the energy for was: 'Please could someone just read my notes?', I was eventually taken through for my injection.

Lying on my side, I watched as the midwife produced and prepared what looked to me like a pretty gigantic needle! She said, 'This one does sting a little.'

The other midwife chipped in, 'She's lying, it can hurt like hell!' Well, at least they weren't sugar-coating it!

In the end, I didn't think it hurt that much at all. It throbbed a little afterwards, and I was encouraged to hold a surgical glove filled with iced water to my own arse cheek (all of the glamour!). It was a quiet Sunday afternoon on the ward, much quieter because of the ongoing Covid-19 precautions, and I looked around at the handful of other women there, some strapped to monitors, others rigged up to drips. I couldn't help but wonder about the circumstances of each one. The road to pregnancy and birth isn't an easy one for so many of us and I thought about the journey they might have been on to get to that ward that day.

The following day's appointment went without a hitch, or any line of questioning that left me wanting the ground to swallow me whole. I was in and out within 15 minutes, the last of my pre-operative injections complete. I hadn't slept a wink that previous night. I wasn't sure if it had been the side effects of the first injection or my pregnancy insomnia ramping up to its final level. Either way, I spent the hours of 2am until 6:30am putting my time to good use and finished reading a book I had wanted to read before I didn't have the time to. The remainder of the day I spent shuffling around (slower than ever now) and getting jobs done in the house, plus enjoying a long afternoon nap – which now felt like a way of life as well as a rite of passage in these final weeks.

The last hurdle would be the following morning, back at the hospital. I was required to have a blood test, an MRSA swab and a Covid swab, all at the drive-through centre, as part of the final preparations for surgery. The midwife who did all three was lovely and I really felt for her sitting out in her pop-up tent at the back of the hospital waiting for patients to pull up. If I had heard it once, I had heard it a thousand times, but these really were 'unprecedented times'. I, for one, really couldn't wait for some precedented times to be back on the cards! The tests were over in a flash and that was it, the last part of the puzzle. I drove away thinking all I needed to do in the next 48 hours was get the washing finished and finally pack my bags. *Then* we would be ready to go.

Later that day, all of the best-laid plans were blown out of the water. As I walked across the kitchen after dinner that evening towards the back doors to let Boris out for an evening wee in the garden, I suddenly felt a sharp pain, coupled with a gush. I looked to the floor and saw a pool of blood. I went to scream and no sound came out.

Frozen to the spot, I grasped for the edge of a chair to cling to as I called out Nico's name. I could hear the chatter from his work colleagues from the room above; he was still working upstairs. I called and called, shouting as loud as I could.

He appeared at the door, calling to me as he arrived, 'Elle, what is it? I'm still working, it's really . . . Oh fuck.' His face looked in horror as he caught sight of me and then of the floor around me.

'What do I do?'

'Grab my phone, call the delivery suite,' I yelled.

The urgency of the situation suddenly hit me as I called instructions to him. This was serious. It felt it and it looked it. My stomach felt tight and motionless as I grasped it, crossing my legs to stop the blood dripping to the floor. Within minutes, having received instructions from the midwives, Nico was on the phone to the ambulance service.

An ambulance was on its way but the call operator stayed on the line. I could hear him on loudspeaker giving instructions to my husband to lay me on the floor, onto my side, to remove my clothes from the waist down and see if he could see an umbilical cord, or even the baby's head?! He kept asking Nico to ask me how I was feeling. I remember very little of that 35-minute wait for the ambulance but I remember how I answered that question: 'I don't care about me, I only care about the baby. Please tell them to hurry up.'

As I lay there, shaking on the floor, tears rolling down my cheeks and my husband squeezing my hand, I couldn't feel the baby moving. I closed my eyes and tried to focus on it, breathing deeply and willing to feel movement. Everything felt like it stood completely still as I lay there.

The ambulance crew arrived; I heard them asking Nico all of the relevant questions. 'How many weeks is she?', 'How old is she?', 'How much blood has she lost?' The list seemed endless. I just wanted to get out of there and get to hospital. After a brief assessment I was straight into the back of the ambulance, no bags packed, covered in blood and tears and no clue as to what was happening. A world away from the meticulously planned birth that we had been preparing for.

I didn't say a word for the entirety of the ambulance journey, gesturing only to the paramedic or my husband with a thumbs up when asked to let them know

I was still OK. I stared at the wall of the ambulance as I lay on my side, still clutching my tummy. I was repeating to myself, *Please, not again. Please be OK. Please.* I don't know who I was pleading with in those minutes between home and the hospital – the baby, the universe perhaps? I just know I have never been so scared in my life and it's no exaggeration to say that I honestly thought it was a certainty that one of us was going to die.

The siren was deafening and the blue lights flashed in my eyes even with them tightly shut. It felt like my worst nightmare was coming true, all over again. I could feel Nico's hand on my shoulder as he kept repeating his own mantra: 'It's OK, you're going to be OK.' It was as though if he said it enough, he might start to believe it, but I could see the fear on his face as they wheeled me out of the ambulance and along the corridor to the lift.

The moment the lift doors opened and we were onto the floor of the delivery suite, it was as though time went from slow-motion to fast-forward. It felt like being in a scene from *Casualty* as they crashed me through the double doors and into the maternity wing. Suddenly about five or so new faces were above me, all wearing masks and telling me their names.

We were in a side room before I could understand what was happening and a mask had been placed around my face too. It was as if everyone was shouting to be heard through their masks – I suppose in case I was in shock or couldn't understand what was happening. They strapped the baby monitor straps around me as Nico stood behind the midwife, holding his breath.

'I'm going to check the baby,' she said, turning the monitor towards her and readjusting the straps. There was look of relief on her face, on everyone's faces, as a heartbeat came pumping out around the room. In that moment I could breathe once more. I was sobbing again but this time it was sheer relief. 'The baby is OK, it's OK,' I repeated to Nico. The baby was OK, but I was still bleeding.

At that moment the doors to the room opened again but this time a familiar face appeared. My consultant stood there in scrubs. I have never in my life been so pleased or relieved to see another human being. 'Oh, thank god!' I yelled (far too loud, I'm sure) as I clocked her. My husband looked equally thankful.

'Even the best-laid plans . . .' were her first words to us. I couldn't help but laugh. I felt myself break into a smile for the first time that night. She was here, I felt safe. It *was* going to be OK. After a quick examination and a chat with the midwives, she came to the side of the bed and said something along the lines of: 'You're still bleeding, we need to keep the baby safe. Babies come when they come, so let's get this one out now shall we?'

A midwife returned to the room and threw a set of scrubs towards my husband, saying, 'You had better get these on.'

'We're having a baby. Now. *Now*?' I said as I looked to her and then to Nico.

'Yes. I'll leave the team to get you ready and the anaesthetist will be in to see you in a minute. I'll see you in theatre shortly.'

I had absolutely no idea what time it was. I asked Nico for my phone, one of the few things he had managed to grab on the way out of the door. It was already gone 9:30pm. I had no idea where the last two hours had gone. It felt like only a matter of minutes had passed by the time the anaesthetist had been to see us and I was already donning my old friends, the surgical stockings and gown (that the very kind midwife had helped me into whilst I was wriggling on the bed, still covered in blood and hanging on to my last shred of dignity). This was it. We were ready.

I was asked if I thought I could walk through to the theatre. I could, and I wanted to. Still dripping blood, I nervously shuffled along the corridor, held and helped along by the midwife and my husband. We were on our way to meet our baby and it all felt beyond surreal. I was saying things to Nico like, 'I haven't done the ironing!' and 'The state of the house when your parents arrive, it's awful!' His parents, who were only a short distance away from us, had made their way straight to our house to look after Boris until mine arrived and had kindly offered to gather up the few things I had begun to pack and bring them straight to the hospital for us.

When I look back now, I think my obsession over those little irrelevant things – like ironing and the state of the floors in our house after I had bled all over them – were my mind's desperate attempts to remove myself from the current situation that we found ourselves in. To focus on the inconsequential things that I could try to control and not on the only thing that should matter right now, the thing I had been building up to for the entire year so far. I knew that within the next 45 minutes our baby would be here, whereas earlier that night I'd thought I still had another 48 hours to prepare.

As I reached the door of the theatre and saw my consultant and her team awaiting my arrival on the other side, I couldn't help but cast my mind back to the moment I had walked out of that last scan appointment and joked about this little one staying put until the time we had planned for their birth. It turned out that this little person had decided they would arrive in (and at) their own sweet time!

I'd love to say that I recall the exact details of how the next part played out, but overcome by emotion (and drugs!) I imagine my recollection might differ to that of anyone else who was in the room that night. So, I'll tell this as best I can remember and hope if anyone who was were to read this, they might remember it in the same way . . .

I was sitting upright on the side of a bed that was raised up high, my back to the friendly anaesthetist who had already exchanged some great banter with my husband and me (very much needed and welcome given the current circumstances!). The room was the brightest I had ever been in, white with light. It dawned on me that though I had been in so many operating theatres in recent years, I had never been in one awake. Everyone around us wore scrubs and masks, some with face visors and goggles too (#CovidTimes). The room felt both calm and controlled – in fact, there was an overwhelming sense of both. People were running through checklists and checking implements before the show began.

I don't know how I had expected to feel. Truth be told, I had never actually allowed myself to think this far ahead, to this moment. But it felt almost as though the excitement was beginning to outweigh the fear, finally, after months of torment and agonising anxiety. I just felt excited to hold our baby in my arms. It took a few attempts to get the needle in my back correctly, but as soon as they got it in I was swiftly shuffled around onto my back and onto the bed before it really kicked in. They tested whether it had taken full effect with an icy cold spray on my shoulder, then spraying upwards from my feet to determine when I could feel it cold against my skin. I could feel my heart pumping in my chest as the curtain was put in place at waist level. Nico sat beside me next, at the head of the bed, squeezing my shoulder with a mixture of excitement and nerves. The lists were still being checked and so was I.

'Are you feeling OK?' asked a doctor.

I suddenly wasn't. I felt hot and dizzy, like I was struggling to breathe.

'Actually, no.'

I knew this was down to my blood pressure having dropped and potentially to me having eaten only a few hours beforehand.

'It's OK, I can give you something to help with that,' replied the anaesthetist.

With that, something else was injected into my cannula as I was tipped up into a different position and people began fanning my face. Within a few moments, I felt a little less like the world was about to end and more like I was back in the room with everyone else. I counted five, six – maybe more – faces above and around me. Machines beeped and I got a sense that proceedings were imminent before I heard the familiar voice of my consultant.

'Eleanor, before we start, who would you like to tell you what you have? Nico?'

All along she had known who was in there, boy or girl, and we were a matter of minutes away from knowing too.

'No,' I replied. 'If it's OK, we'd like you to tell us?'

There was no way I was going to let her come on this ride with us (and what a hell of a ride it had been to this point) and not take that final moment of glory. I wanted to thank her for everything she had done but

I knew that the words 'thank you' would never feel enough.

Music played around the operating theatre as they began. It felt so relaxed; I could hear people merrily humming along to 'Hey Soul Sister', a song that had landed on my playlist that we had also walked out of the church to on our wedding day. Its familiarity and happy memories made me feel safe and calm.

I turned to Nico, who was staring intently towards the direction of the curtain and intermittently at me to give a reassuring smile. He already looked as though he had tears in his eyes. I could feel my eyes prickling too.

'You're going to feel some tugging now,' said a head which came to our side of the curtain.

They weren't wrong. It was the most bizarre sensation as they pulled and pushed the baby down. I could just about see the head and shoulders of the doctor doing the pushing – she almost looked as though she was jumping up and down on a trampoline to push the baby into the right position for exit.

'Almost there,' came from the kind midwife who we had met at the beginning of our evening. She had stayed next to me throughout and was still here, smiling and willing us on.

Then, a moment of silence and I held my breath. It felt as though everyone else held their breath too.

Not for long, as within seconds the room was filled with loud and wonderful screams. Not from me, for once, but from a tiny human on the other side of the curtain. As it lowered, I saw my consultant's face as she cradled and gestured this tiny person towards us. Even with her mask on I could see from her eyes that she was smiling.

'You have a little girl.'

In a blur, the cord was clamped, she was checked by paediatricians who had been waiting, in light of our history. I'll never forget the words from one of the doctors who came right next to my face and said, 'The paediatricians are leaving now, because your baby is perfectly well.'

Perfectly well. A screaming baby. Two things I had longed for, had dreamed of for so long. As they pulled my gown back and placed her at the top of my chest, her skin to mine, I watched as her eyes, already open, gazed up at my face. She sucked my cheek as my tears rolled down them. McFly's 'All About You' filled the operating theatre as doctors and midwifes congratulated us.

'A little girl. A healthy little girl,' I repeated over and over to Nico as he put his face up next to mine and we both stared back at her in complete wonderment. In that moment, it was as if everything that had come before just melted away, because we were here, with her, and that was all that mattered.

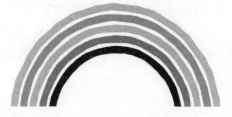

Chapter 21

To the Girl in the Mirror

I DON'T GIVE ADVICE ABOUT FERTILITY, ABOUT LOSS, OR ABOUT MUCH, REALLY. I don't feel qualified to – because I'm not. I'm just someone who went through some things and decided to write those things down in the hope that, one day, they might help someone else, someone going through something similar, to feel less alone. But I have often wondered, what would I say to myself? The girl who stood and looked in the mirror at 39 weeks pregnant with her first child, over four and a half years ago, and took a photo in excited anticipation of the journey ahead of her. The one who didn't have a clue about the things to come or quite how much of a bump in the road she was about to encounter . . .

❦

Dear Elle,

I know you're excited. I can see that on your smiling face. You have been so excited for this baby to arrive and so you should be. I'm not quite sure how to even tell you this, as I look at you here, but things aren't going to turn out how you're imagining right now. The next few weeks will turn into a nightmare, your worst nightmare, and the next four years will be harder than anything you could have pictured. You'll meet and hold your beautiful son and then you'll have to say goodbye. You'll feel like your heart is shattering into a thousand pieces and like you might break into pieces. But you won't, I promise you.

You'll meet new friends who will understand your heartbreak only too well and you'll lose some along the way. There will be times that you feel like no one understands what you're truly feeling, and like those feelings are going to engulf you and stop you from carrying on, but they won't. I promise that too.

You'll want to try again, try to give Teddy a brother or sister, try to live the motherhood you had dreamed of instead of the reality you find yourself caught in. You'll discover that won't be the road you expected it to be either. You'll experience loss again and again. You'll begin to wonder whether the universe might ever cut you some slack but you'll keep hoping that it might. You'll feel as though you are putting your body, mind and heart through more than they were ever meant to take on this quest to be the mum you had hoped to be. And it will feel like a never-ending quest, I can tell you that much.

It will feel as though everyone around you can achieve so easily something you can only dream of. You'll start to feel left out, left behind and left with no hope, living in a limbo land that you're desperate to escape. But there is hope, that I can promise you. You'll start to dislike yourself when you feel mad, jealous or resentful at others for making it look so effortless. You'll feel like your body is letting you down and like you're letting the side down. You're not.

You'll try everything, and I mean everything, to make this happen. There will be no 'cure' you won't entertain and you'll guess that others around you are tolerating each new 'thing' as it comes along. You'll drink a LOT of beetroot juice (and you'll still fucking hate it) and fill out more paperwork than you ever thought was possible. The tears you'll cry could probably fill a bath tub, or a swimming pool, perhaps even an ocean? It will feel relentless and, at times, you will want to throw in the towel and just start living life again because it hurts your heart too much to carry on and it begins to feel like it's hurting the people you love the most too. There will be moments that you want to scream and cry simultaneously: both will make you feel better in equal measure, if only momentarily. You'll make plans that you fear will never come to fruition and dream of things you are scared you'll never live to see. All the while trying so hard to visualise them in your mind, so that one day they might just come true.

Despite all of this, you won't give up and you won't stop hoping. One day, when you least expect it, magic will happen. You'll worry every day that it still won't be your time. You expect catastrophe and heartbreak around every corner because that's what you've trained yourself to prepare for. You'll make a wish every day that this time dreams might just come true. The road will feel dark and long and often lonely. And then one day your sun will shine again.

One day, after those years and tears and heartbreak, you'll find yourself in a single moment that will feel as though you've travelled a full circle in time. On a Tuesday afternoon, you'll stand in the autumn sunshine in a park you walked through every day in those early weeks and months of grief, a place your feet trod over and over during the toughest of times. You'll realise that you're in the exact spot where you stood a little over four years ago, after you had walked alone past a group of mums with new-born babies, as they chattered about you, knowing your loss and yet not saying hello. Tears streaming down your face as you hid as best you could behind your sunglasses before you hurried on.

On that Tuesday, you'll stand in that spot again and look up, through the leaves on the trees, and squint through the late afternoon sunshine to the spire of the church where you held your *precious son's funeral. Then you'll look down to your daughter's face, her cheek pressed to your chest as she sleeps peacefully in her carrier. Another mum will pass you with her pram and say cheerily, 'She's beautiful, how old?' You'll chatter and then say goodbye. She won't know how much that moment meant to you. You'll feel a sense of complete redemption, of forgiveness for those who never understood, or who couldn't find the right words to say. You'll look again at your daughter's sleeping face and, feeling your heart swell beyond anything you've felt before, those tears will roll down your face once more.*

That day, you'll finally realise that it was, always, meant to be her.

Whatever happens, you'll get to that moment. Exactly where you need to be. And your sun will shine again, I promise.

Elle x

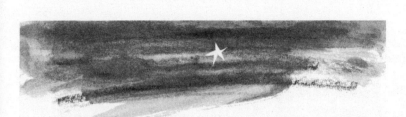

And finally it
was our turn,
to feel your
warm body
against my heart,
to belong to
each other,
to be your
mum.

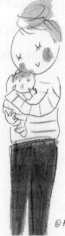

©Anna Lewis - Sketchy Muma.

Useful Stuff

THERE ARE MANY THINGS THAT HAVE HELPED ME ON MY WAY ALONG THIS ROAD: CHARITIES, SUPPORT NETWORKS, BOOKS AND MORE. I am not saying these are for everyone but you might just find something here that helps you too . . .

Books
Fertile, Emma Cannon
The Baby-Making Bible, Emma Cannon
It Starts with The Egg, Rebecca Fett
The IVF Diet, Zita West
Inconceivable, Julia Indichova
Life After Baby Loss, Nicola Gaskin

Journals

The Bees Knees Journal, Kelly Terranova
A positivity journal created by Kelly Terranova in the wake of her own family's heartbreak (her mum's diagnosis of Huntington's Disease). Kelly has channelled her positive energy into a daily journal for people to reflect on their days. These journals helped me immensely over three years and encouraged me to try to think less about living from cycle to cycle, or treatment dates to treatment dates. It definitely helped to alter my focus and appreciate the small things in each day that make us smile. www.thebeesknees.co

Fertility and Trying to Conceive Support
Zita West
www.zitawestclinic.com
Emma Cannon
www.emmacannon.co.uk
Fertility Network
www.fertilitynetworkuk.org
Big Fat Negative (podcast and community)
www.bigfatnegative.com
Alice Rose, Fertility Life Raft podcast
Cat Strawbridge, The Finally Pregnant podcast and community
www.catstrawbridge.com

Loss Support
Tommy's
www.tommys.org
ARC (Antenatal Results and Choices)
www.arc-uk.org
The Miscarriage Association
www.miscarriageassociation.org.uk
The Ectopic Pregnancy Trust
www.ectopic.org.uk/
Our Missing Peace (there to help everyone who has been affected by the death of a child)
www.ourmissingpeace.org
Sands (stillbirth and neonatal death charity)
www.sands.org.uk
Teddy's Wish (funding research into the causes of baby loss and providing hope for grieving families)
www.teddyswish.org
Mariposa Trust, Saying Goodbye (providing information and support to anyone who has suffered the loss of a baby)
www.sayinggoodbye.org

Acknowledgements

Once again, there are so many people I need to thank for making this book happen. Firstly, to every single person who read *Ask Me His Name* and took the time to read about Teddy. Without you, there would undoubtedly not have been a book two. To the readers of my blog and Instagram posts; thank you for always engaging in and continuing the conversation around loss and fertility struggles. It always brings me great comfort to know that we are going though this together.

Lauren, where do I start? You have, once again, been a guide, a friend and someone who catches the ball when I have most definitely dropped it. Thank you for listening to all of the lengthy voice notes when I didn't have the capacity to use email, and for always knowing the right thing to say when I was struggling. This would not have happened without you.

Thank you to Beth, for believing in this book. For allowing me to write an unfiltered account of loss and fertility struggles, with far too many 'fucks' thrown in. Thank you for your patience, kindness and guidance. P.S. I am sorry the cover took so long . . . again.

Thank you to Louise, Angie and Gretchen for helping me along this journey and becoming friends, who wanted this as much as I did. Emma, for your wise words, wisdom and calm. You showed me there could be a way if I believed there could be. I believe in miracles and magic because of you.

Thank you to my mum, Carol, for her love and support. For proof-reading and spell-checking at a time I was left (quite literally) holding the baby. I think we can safely say that if there are any mistakes in here, then I can blame you? I could not have done this without you. I love you.

Thank you to Rachel, Vanessa, Zara and Sophie. This book is what it is because of your contributions. Thank you for your openness, honesty and bravery. I hope it is a book that does so much more than just recount one story and one outcome. I hope it will bring something to many, and that will be because of you all.

Nico, thank you. The last five years have brought times that I never could have imagined, and there is no one else who I could have faced those things with. Thank you for picking me up, holding my hand and always helping me to smile again.

To my friends (you know who you are!). Thank you for listening when I just needed someone to listen. Thank you for the hugs, the chats, the kind words and for never trying to 'fix it' for me. I promise I will always be there for you all when you need me, too.

Lastly, to *all* of the doctors, nurses and midwives who helped us along this ride. Donna, for staying with me when I needed you the most. Alison, for staying late to operate on me because you knew how scared I was. Georgina and Suzy, for always going above and beyond in helping me. Jules, for knowing how to make me laugh and smile at each scan, whether it was bad news or good. Rebecca, for being there when I had given up hope. Sally and Michelle, for holding my hand along the way and helping me to believe there could be a happy outcome. Astrid, for being there to share in our happiest moment and for asking about Teddy. Renata, I cannot even find the words – thank you will never seem like enough for all you have done for us; but from the bottom of my heart, thank you.